Advances in Human Clinical Nutrition

Advances in Human Clinical Nutrition

Edited by

Joseph J. Vitale, ScD, MD

Selwyn A. Broitman, PhD

Boston University School of Medicine

Boston, MA

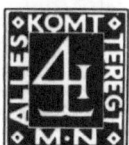

1982
MARTINUS NIJHOFF PUBLISHERS
THE HAGUE / BOSTON / LONDON

Distributors for all countries outside North America

Kluwer Academic Publishers Group
Distribution Center
P.O. Box 322
3300 AH Dordrecht
The Netherlands

Medicine is an ever-changing science. As new research and clinical experience broaden our knowledge, changes in treatment and drug therapy are required. The editors and the publisher of this work have made every effort to ensure that the treatment and drug dosage schedules herein are accurate and in accord with standards accepted at the time of publication. Readers are advised, however, to check the product information sheet included in the package of each drug they plan to administer to be certain that changes have not been made in the recommended dose or in the indications and contraindications for administration. This recommendation is of particular importance in regard to new or infrequently used drugs.

Joint edition published by

MARTINUS NIJHOFF PUBLISHERS
P.O. Box 566, 2501 CN The Hague, The Netherlands

and

John Wright • PSG Inc
545 Great Road
Littleton, Massachusetts 01460, U.S.A.

This volume is listed in the Library of Congress Cataloging in Publication Data

ISBN-13: 978-94-009-8292-5   e-ISBN-13: 978-94-009-8290-1
DOI: 10.1007/978-94-009-8290-1

Softcover reprint of the hardcover 1st edition 1982

CONTRIBUTORS

Ronald A. Arky, MD
Professor of Medicine
Harvard Medical School

William R. Beisel, MD
Scientific Advisor
US Army Medical Research Institute
 of Infectious Diseases
Frederick, Md

George L. Blackburn, MD, PhD
Associate Professor of Surgery
Harvard Medical School

John M. Carper, MD
Associate Professor of Pediatrics
Boston University
 School of Medicine

Angel Cordano, MD, MPH
Associate Director
Nutritional Division
Mead Johnson & Company
Evansville, Ind

Hector F. DeLuca, PhD
Professor and Chairman
Department of Biochemistry
University of Wisconsin
 Medical School

Richard J. Elkort, MD
Assistant Professor of Surgery
Boston University
 School of Medicine

Ophilia James, MD
Assistant Professor of Pediatrics
Boston University
 School of Medicine

David Kritchevsky, PhD
Associate Director
Wistar Institute of Anatomy
 and Biology
Philadelphia, Pa

Neal S. LeLeiko, MD, PhD
Assistant Professor of Pediatrics
Mount Sinai School of Medicine
New York, NY

Baltej S. Maini, MD
Research Associate
Cancer Research Institute
New England Deaconess Hospital
Boston, Mass

Kathleen J. Motil, MD, PhD
Assistant in Medicine
Children's Hospital Medical Center
Boston, Mass

Robert E. Olson, MD, PhD
Professor and Chairman
Department of Biochemistry
St. Louis University
 School of Medicine

Eileen Ouellette, MD
Assistant Professor of Neurology
Harvard Medical School

Jon A. Story, PhD
Associate Professor of Nutrition
Purdue University

John W. Suttie, PhD
Professor of Biochemistry
University of Wisconsin
 Medical School

Joseph J. Vitale, ScD, MD
Director of Nutrition
 Education Programs
Professor of Pathology
Associate Dean
 for International Health
Boston University
 School of Medicine

Esther Wender, MD
Associate Professor of Pediatrics
University of Utah
College of Medicine

Steven H. Zeisel, MD
Assistant Professor of Nutrition
Massachusetts Institute
 of Technology

EDITORS

Joseph J. Vitale, ScD, MD
Director of Nutrition Education Programs
Professor of Pathology
Associate Dean for International Health
Boston University School of Medicine

Selwyn A. Broitman, PhD
Professor of Microbiology and Nutritional Sciences
Boston University School of Medicine

CONTENTS

PREFACE

Boston University School of Medicine has established a series of Medical Education Programs in Nutrition held each summer since 1975. These deal with controversies in human clinical nutrition. The subjects have covered various topics, including those dealing with the relationships between diet and heart disease, diet and cancer, breast versus bottle-feeding, and dietary fiber and disease. Other noncontroversial topics were also covered at these conferences; they were discussed simply to bring to the attention of the health professional new happenings in nutritional research. These topics dealt with the relationships of nutrition to immune function, to neurotransmitters, to infection, to obesity, and to chemotherapy.

This text is a compilation of selected manuscripts of interest to the health professional in the area of human clinical nutrition.

Whatever success this text enjoys is in no small way due to the administrative and editorial efforts of our administrative assistant, Mrs Geraldine Rankin — our sincere thanks.

Joseph J. Vitale, ScD, MD
Selwyn A. Broitman, PhD

Advances in Human Clinical Nutrition

1 Issues and Advances in Human and Clinical Nutrition

Joseph J. Vitale, ScD, MD

As any medical historian will testify, the history of medicine is replete with controversies, many of which are related to nutrition. Webster defines the word controversy as a "discussion of a question in which opposing opinions clash; debate, disputation; a quarrel or a dispute; controversy connotes a disagreement of lengthy duration of a matter of some weight or importance."[1] This definition, while adequate for most purposes, is inadequate for others, since it makes no reference to what should or should not be accepted in a discussion of a question. When should the discussion include theoretical considerations, or universally accepted or proven facts? If we allowed only the latter, there would be no controversy nor would any conference ever have been planned. If on the other hand we allow theoretical considerations, we should insist, I believe, that they be connected by a series of simple logical steps to generally accepted knowledge, and that they be put to the best possible experimental test. For example, antihistamines help mitigate effects of the common cold. High doses of vitamin C have antihistaminic effects; therefore high doses of vitamin C may be beneficial to individuals with colds — logical! To carry this further and believe that high doses of vitamin C may prevent the common cold would be illogical.

1

The President's Biological Research Panel in 1976 addressed itself to the lags between initial discovery and clinical application in cardiovascular-pulmonary medicine and surgery. The panelists used the neurophysiologist's definition, whereby a lag is a time interval between a stimulus and an appropriate response. More specifically, they defined lag as the number of years between an initial discovery for any purpose, including knowledge gained for the sake of knowledge, and its effective clinical application. Considering the lag times between the 132 discoveries listed and the first clinical application in just this one specialty, cardiovascular-pulmonary medicine and surgery, 43 were applied in less than 10 years; 27 in 10 to 24 years; 39 in 25 to 49 years; 18 in 50 to 99 years; and 5 in 100 years or more. The authors listed 17 causes of lags and there are probably more; these vary with the century or generation and with prevailing attitudes toward science, religion, medicine, and morality; with then-current political, ethical, sociologic, and economic factors; with one's perception of the knowledge base existing at the time; and with the availability of facilities and resources for animal or clinical investigation, and their restrictions. Opposing opinions and controversies arise from such causes and have inherent in their expression, among other things, personal attitudes, feelings, and vested interests. These and other factors undoubtedly are involved in the generally accepted phenomenon of the resistance to "scientific discovery" on the part of scientists; one should hasten to add, with justifiable cause in many cases. It would be interesting to have available a list of discoveries that turned out to be no discovery at all.

Controversies related to nutrition have existed in the past, they exist today, and I suspect that they will continue to exist. It took over 35 years to settle the controversy that beriberi was not an infectious disease. I feel certain that most of us would consider this to be related to the prevailing attitudes toward science at the time and the then-current feelings about the pathogenesis of disease. Any suggestion, during the time of Pasteur and Koch, that a disease state was due to anything other than a positive toxic, or infectious agent, would have been sacrilegious. It took almost another 35 to 40 years to convince many people that, indeed, disease could be brought about by the absence of certain factors, and the award of the Nobel prize to both Hopkins and Eijkman firmly established the basis for the etiology of deficiency states. Needless to say, it was through appropriate experimental procedures, and through animal and human experimentation, that the question of whether beriberi was an infectious disease or a deficiency disease was finally settled; the controversy was over with the observation that the deficiency of thiamine caused beriberi. The lag period between Eijkman's observations in chickens in the late 1800s and the discovery of thiamine might have taken longer if the question pertaining to the cause of beriberi was settled by theoretical considerations alone.

Rickets is associated with vitamin D deficiency, and scurvy with vitamin C deficiency. A great deal of work, time, and effort went into these discoveries; and certainly many controversies were involved between the initial observations of clinical scurvy or rickets and the identification of their causes.

While there may be deficiency states yet to be uncovered, major controversies in nutrition in the 1970s seemed to center around patterns of feeding (ie, breast versus bottle), nutritional excesses, and dietary aberrations.

With regard to breast- versus bottle-feeding, nonnutritionists as well as nutritionists have become involved in this controversy. Recently there has been a great deal of interest in the manner in which companies promote their products, particularly those in the infant food industry, and about the health hazards of bottle-feeding in contrast to breast-feeding. One of the problems with nutrition is that people too often become righteous in their pronouncements about nutrition and leave reasoning to the wind. There is no controversy as to whether or not a mother should breast-feed. If there are no contraindications, most health professionals believe that the mother should breast-feed. Rather, the controversy that does exist concerns itself with the question of whether breast milk delivered in a clean environment offers any better opportunities for growth or any better protection to the infant against infectious disease processes than do breast-milk substitutes. All are agreed that there is a need for a breast-milk substitute in many underdeveloped areas, where the mother is unable to continue breast-feeding because of her own poor nutritional status. But the question remains, does breast milk in an aseptic environment offer any advantages over bottle-feeding to the infant in terms of growth or susceptibility to infection or to diseases later in life? Several of our contributors to this text will deal with this question. The readers are left to draw their own conclusions regarding the issues as to whether feeding in a clean environment offers any advantage over bottle-feeding to the infant.

Volumes have been written about nutritional excesses, and it is likely that volumes more will be written in the future. In discussing aberrations we must remember that the word means "a departure from what is right, true, or correct, or a deviation from the normal or typical."[2] With regard to nutritional excesses we are on much firmer ground in dealing with excess calories and the associated problem of obesity, than we are with excesses of specific nutrients or with dietary aberrations, or with what is right, true, correct, or the optimal diet.

Once nutritional requirements are met, we move out of the area of deficiency states into the unknown, in terms of optimal nutrition and its relation to health and disease. In recent years a great deal has been said and written about the optimal diet in terms of the quality and quantity of various dietary components such as fat, fiber, and carbohydrate with respect to several public health problems, including cancer and heart disease. There are those who feel that diets high in saturated fats are indeed aberrations since they may predispose to cardiovascular disease, while others feel that diets high in unsaturated fats are dietary aberrations in that they may predispose to malignancy.

Olson, one of the contributors to this text, in his W.O. Atwater Memorial Lecture,[3] listed the various genetic and nutritional determinants for 13 diseases. I think he would agree that, in addition to genetic and nutritional determinants, there may be other determinants, such as those found in the environment, which may interact with genetic and nutritional determinants either in an additive or a synergistic fashion to complicate the role of any one determinant in the pathogenesis of disease. To cite a few examples, in sickle cell anemia and hemophilia, the genetic determinant accounts for practically 100% of the illness, and no nutritional control is possible. At the other end of the spectrum are diseases like scurvy, rickets, or beriberi, in which the disease is almost entirely controlled by nutritional and/or environmental manipulations. Somewhere between these two extremes lie two major diseases, atherosclerosis and cancer, which account for a great deal of the mortality and morbidity seen in our country. The major problem in attempting to prescribe the optimal diet, or in discussing aberrations in diet, relates to the multiple-etiologic aspect of disease. Heart disease and cancer are intermediate on the scale of genetic and nutritional determinants and hence may never be totally controllable by dietary intervention, eg, by the quality of fat, carbohydrate, or fiber in the diet. It should be stressed that diet is a conglomeration of not only nutrients, both essential and nonessential, but of food additives, preservatives, etc, some of which may be carcinogenic or atherogenic. There is little evidence, experimental or otherwise, that any nutrient excess or any nutrient deficiency per se has ever resulted in cancer, myocardial infarction, or sudden death in animals or humans.

Most of the common diseases, particularly cancer and atherosclerosis, are probably multifactorial in origin involving not only nutrients but perhaps co-carcinogens or co-atherogens, which may be elements of the diet. Scurvy, pellagra, and goiter, on the other hand, do result from aberrations in the diet and/or environment; they may be primary or induced deficiency states and they can be totally controlled by diet. With regard to the associated risk factors, obesity and diabetes, people talk about obesity as they do about health, as though it were some known and measurable quantity. Yet most people agree that its meaning is elusive; the use of the word obesity contrasts with any clear, distinct, or generally acceptable definition. The fundamental question is the extent to which excessive fat stores impair health. For an excellent discussion about obesity, in contrast to overweight, as a risk factor, the reader is referred to an article by Mann.[4] It appears that weight exceeding ideal by as much as 20% may not place an individual at risk to known diseases. However, morbid obesity, where weight exceeds 30% of ideal weight, may place the individual at risk for cardiovascular disease, diabetes, and hypertension.

Notwithstanding the differing opinions among nutritionists, the Select Committee on Nutrition and Human Needs of the US Senate has urged the adoption of the American Heart Association's Program of Dietary Prevention, not only for atherosclerosis and its complications but also for cancer and diabetes. These dietary goals for the United States published in February 1977 and revised in December 1977 have been the center of intense controversy (Appendix).

Depending on one's outlook and attitudes, there are some who apparently agree with Sir Edward Mellanby, a noted nutritionist, who once said: "No nutritional policy adopted by governments can be wrong if it places the health and needs of the community as its first and guiding principal." Sir Edward obviously had more faith in the wisdom of his government than some of us have in ours. One could only agree with Sir Edward if the nutritional policy was based on scientific facts and not nurtured by vested interests. The major thrust of the report on dietary goals was that, if the American public modified their food intake they could not only control their heart disease but perhaps prevent it. The implication was the same for cancer, ie, a change from present dietary habits to those that would follow the dietary goals would prevent cancer or certainly reduce its incidence significantly. Much has been written concerning the dietary goals; perhaps the best critical review was written by Harper.[6]

Many nutritionists who oppose the thrust of the dietary goals argue that if one followed them, they might be jumping "from a frying pan into the fire." Indeed, a number of studies have now been published that suggest that changes from diets high in saturated fats to those relatively high in unsaturated fats have had no impact on the course of cardiovascular disease, and indeed may have left the individual at greater risk to cancer.[7,8] It is interesting now that the proponents of the dietary goals have modified their stand; more recently they have begun to "tout the no-risk aspects of the dietary goals rather that emphasizing their ability to prevent disease.[9] In fairness to the proponents of the dietary goals, however, the reader is referred to an article by Hegsted[10] in which he states his own position and defends the dietary goals. Dr. Hegsted is quoted as saying: "The question to be asked is not why we change our diet, but why not? What are the risks associated with eating less meat, less fat, less cholesterol, less sugar, and less salt? There are none that can be identified and important benefits can be expected."[9] The opposition, of course, says that risks do exist, and that public expectations would be raised needlessly.

It was also of interest to read in the *Dairy Council Digest* about the "virtues" of cholesterol.[11] In a good review of cholesterol metabolism, the Digest points out the essentiality of cholesterol for all cells, extolls the fine feedback mechanisms controlling serum cholesterol levels and, among other things, points out that the cholesterol content of the US diet is much the same today as it was in 1909, about 500 mg per capita per day. As we all know, mortality from cardiovascular disease has been declining for the last ten years or so, notwithstanding insignificant changes in dietary habits or in serum cholesterol levels. Dietary-intervention studies have not been shown to alter mortality rates from cardiovascular disease, and, as we pointed out, some studies have suggested that a switch to diets high in unsaturated fat or to other regimens designed to lower serum cholesterol may be a switch to an increased risk of oncogenesis. Mann has expressed his skepticism about diet-heart relationships,[12] sentiments shared by many of us in nutrition.

We believe that most nutritionists would agree that the best advice one can presently give is: 1) attempt to maintain one's weight as close as possible to that attained at age 25, or to one's ideal weight; 2) improve or optimize physical and emotional well-being; 3) stop smoking; 4) control hypertension and diabetes; and 5) decrease the level of dietary fat as much as possible, increase the level of dietary fiber, and vary the diet to include items from all the various food groups.

The proponents of the dietary goals first led the American public to believe that if the recommendations were followed, we could do much to prevent such diseases as heart disease and cancer. More recently, however, they have switched and now tout "the no-risk aspects of dietary goals."[9] The available evidence suggests that for some this is still an inadequate change of position.

From a global standpoint, although dietary deficiency is definitely at the more serious end of the spectrum, the opposite end, dietary excesses and possible aberrations, may nonetheless contribute to the burden of disease.

APPENDIX

NUTRITION AND YOUR HEALTH

Dietary Guidelines for Americans

What should you eat to stay healthy?

Hardly a day goes by without someone trying to answer that question. Newspapers, magazines, books, radio, and television give us a lot of advice about what foods we should or should not eat. Unfortunately, much of this advice is confusing.

Some of this confusion exists because we don't know enough about nutrition to identify an "ideal diet" for each individual. People differ — and their food needs vary depending on age, sex, body size, physical activity, and other conditions such as pregnancy or illness.

In those chronic conditions where diet may be important — heart attacks, high blood pressure, strokes, dental caries, diabetes, and some forms of cancer — the roles of specific nutrients have not been defined.

Research does seek to find more precise nutritional requirements and to show better the connections between diet and certain chronic diseases.

But today, what advice should you follow in choosing and preparing the best foods for you and your family?

The guidelines below are suggested for most Americans. They do not apply to people who need special diets because of diseases or conditions that interfere with normal nutrition. These people may require special instruction from trained dietitians, in consultation with their own physicians.

These guidelines are intended for people who are already healthy. No guidelines can guarantee health or well-being. Health depends on many things, including heredity, lifestyle, personality traits, mental health and attitudes, and environment, in addition to diet.

Food alone cannot make you healthy. But good eating habits based on moderation and variety can help keep you healthy and even improve your health.

Dietary Guidelines for Americans
- Eat a variety of foods
- Maintain ideal weight
- Avoid too much fat, saturated fat, and cholesterol
- Eat food with adequate starch and fiber
- Avoid too much sugar
- Avoid too much sodium
- If you drink alcohol, do so in moderation

Eat a Variety of Foods

You need about 40 different nutrients to stay healthy. These include vitamins and minerals, as well as amino acids (from proteins), essential fatty acids (from vegetable oils and animal fats), and sources of energy (calories from carbohydrates, proteins, and fats). These nutrients are in the foods you normally eat.

Most foods contain more than one nutrient. Milk, for example, provides proteins, fats, sugars, riboflavin and other B-vitamins, vitamin A, calcium, and phosphorus — among other nutrients.

No single food item supplies all the essential nutrients in the amounts that you need. Milk, for instance, contains very little iron or vitamin C. You should, therefore, eat a variety of foods to assure an adequate diet.

The greater the variety, the less likely you are to develop either a deficiency or an excess of any single nutrient. Variety also reduces your likelihood of being exposed to excessive amounts of contaminants in any single food item.

One way to assure variety and, with it, a well-balanced diet is to select foods each day from each of several major groups: for example, fruits and vegetables; cereals, breads, and grains; meats, poultry, eggs, and fish; dry peas and beans, such as soybeans, kidney beans, lima beans, and black-eyed peas, which are good vegetable sources of protein; and milk, cheese, and yogurt.

Fruits and vegetables are excellent sources of vitamins, especially vitamins C and A. Whole grain and enriched breads, cereals, and grain products provide B-vitamins, iron, and energy. Meats supply protein, fat, iron and other minerals, as well as several vitamins including thiamine and vitamin B_{12}. Dairy products are major sources of calcium and other nutrients.

To Assure Yourself An Adequate Diet — Eat a variety of foods daily, including selections of
- Fruits
- Vegetables
- Whole grain and enriched breads, cereals, and grain products
- Milk, cheese, and yogurt
- Meats, poultry, fish, eggs
- Legumes (dry peas and beans)

There are no known advantages to consuming excess amounts of any nutrient. You will rarely need to take vitamin or mineral supplements if you eat a wide variety of foods. There are a few important exceptions to this general statement:
- *Women in their childbearing years* may need to take iron supplements

to replace the iron they lose with menstrual bleeding. Women who are no longer menstruating should not take iron supplements routinely.

• *Women who are pregnant or who are breastfeeding* need more of many nutrients, especially iron, folic acid, vitamin A, calcium, and sources of energy (calories from carbohydrates, proteins, and fats). Detailed advice should come from their physicians or from dietitians.

• *Elderly or very inactive people* may eat relatively little food. Thus, they should pay special attention to avoiding foods that are high in calories but low in other essential nutrients—for example, fat, oils, alcohol, and sugars.

Infants also have special nutritional needs. Healthy full-term infants should be breast-fed unless there are special problems. The nutrients in human breast milk tend to be digested and absorbed more easily than those in cow's milk. In addition, breast milk may serve to transfer immunity to some diseases from the mother to the infant.

Normally, most babies do not need solid foods until they are 3 to 6 months old. At that time, other foods can be introduced gradually. Prolonged breast or bottlefeeding—without solid foods or supplemental iron—can result in iron deficiency.

You should not add salt or sugar to the baby's foods. Infants do not need these "encouragements"—if they are really hungry. The foods themselves contain enough salt and sugar; extra is not necessary.

To Assure Your Baby An Adequate Diet
- Breastfeed unless there are special problems
- Delay other foods until baby is 3 to 6 months old
- Do not add salt or sugar to baby's food

MAINTAIN IDEAL WEIGHT

If you are too fat, your chances of developing some chronic disorders are increased. Obesity is associated with high blood pressure, increased levels of blood fats (triglycerides) and cholesterol, and the most common type of diabetes. All of these, in turn, are associated with increased risks of heart attacks and strokes. Thus, you should try to maintain "ideal" weight.

But, how do you determine what the ideal weight is for you?

There is no absolute answer. The table on the following page shows "acceptable" ranges for most adults. If you have been obese since childhood, you may find it difficult to reach or to maintain your weight within the acceptable range. For most people, their weight should not be more that it was when they were young adults (20 or 25 years old).

It is not well understood why some people can eat much more than others and still maintain normal weight. However, one thing is definite: to lose weight, you must take in fewer calories than you burn. This means that you must either select foods containing fewer calories or you must increase your activity—or both.

10

Suggested Body Weights

| Height (feet-inches) | Range of Acceptable Weight | |
	Men (pounds)	Women (pounds)
4–10		92-119
4–11		94-122
5–0		96-125
5–1		99-128
5–2	112-141	102-131
5–3	115-144	105-134
5–4	118-148	108-138
5–5	121-152	111-142
5–6	124-156	114-146
5–7	128-161	118-150
5–8	132-166	122-154
5–9	136-170	126-158
5–10	140-174	130-163
5–11	144-179	134-168
6–0	148-184	138-173
6–1	152-189	
6–2	156-194	
6–3	160-199	
6–4	164-204	

NOTE: Height without shoes; weight without clothes.
SOURCE: HEW conference on obesity, 1973.

To Improve Eating Habits
- Eat slowly
- Prepare smaller portions
- Avoid "seconds"

If you need to lose weight, do so gradually. Steady loss of 1 to 2 pounds a week — until you reach your goal — is relatively safe and more likely to be maintained. Long-term success depends upon acquiring new and better habits of eating and exercise. That is perhaps why "crash" diets usually fail in the long run.

Do not try to lose weight too rapidly. Avoid crash diets that are severely restricted in the variety of foods they allow. Diets containing fewer than 800 calories may be hazardous. Some people have developed kidney stones, disturbing psychological changes, and other complications while following such diets. A few people have died suddenly and without warning.

To Lose Weight
- Increase physical activity
- Eat less fat and fatty foods

- Eat less sugar and sweets
- Avoid too much alcohol

Gradual increase of everyday physical activities like walking or climbing stairs can be very helpful. The chart below gives the calories used per hour in different activities.

Approximate Energy Expenditure by a 150 Pound Person in Various Activites

Activity	Calories per hour
Lying down or sleeping	80
Sitting	100
Driving an automobile	120
Standing	140
Domestic work	180
Walking, 2-1/2 mph	210
Bicycling, 5-1/2 mph	210
Gardening	220
Golf; lawn mowing, power mower	250
Bowling	270
Walking, 3-3/4 mph	300
Swimming, 1/4 mph	300
Square dancing, volleyball: roller skating	350
Wood chopping or sawing	400
Tennis	420
Skiing, 10 mph	600
Squash and handball	600
Bicycling, 13 mph	660
Running, 10 mph	900

SOURCE: Based on material prepared by Robert E. Johnson, M.D., Ph.D., and colleagues, University of Illinois.

A pound of body fat contains 3500 calories. To lose 1 pound of fat, you will need to burn 3500 calories more than you consume. If you burn 500 calories more a day than you consume, you will lose 1 pound of fat a week. Thus, if you normally burn 1700 calories a day, you can theoretically expect to lose a pound of fat each week if you adhere to a 1200-calorie-per-day diet.

Do not attempt to reduce your weight below the acceptable range. Severe weight loss may be associated with nutrient deficiencies, menstrual irregularities, infertility, hair loss, skin changes, cold intolerance, severe constipation, psychiatric disturbances, and other complications.

If you lose weight suddenly or for unknown reasons, see a physician. Unexplained weight loss may be an early clue to an unsuspected underlying disorder.

Avoid Too Much Fat, Saturated Fat, and Cholesterol

If you have a high blood cholesterol level, you have a greater chance of having a heart attack. Other factors can also increase your risk of heart attack — high blood pressure and cigarette smoking, for example — but high blood cholesterol is clearly a major dietary risk indicator.

Populations like ours with diets high in saturated fats and cholesterol tend to have high blood cholesterol levels. Individuals within these populations usually have greater risks of having heart attacks than people eating low-fat, low-cholesterol diets.

Eating extra saturated fat and cholesterol will increase blood cholesterol levels in most people. However, there are wide variations among people — related to heredity and the way each person's body uses cholesterol.

Some people can consume diets high in saturated fats and cholesterol and still keep normal blood cholesterol levels. Other people, unfortunately, have high blood cholesterol levels even if they eat low-fat, low cholesterol diets.

There is controversy about what recommendations are appropriate for healthy Americans. But for the U.S. population *as a whole*, reduction in our current intake of total fat, saturated fat, and cholesterol is sensible. This suggestion is especially appropriate for people who have high blood pressure or who smoke.

The recommendations are not meant to prohibit the use of any specific food item or to prevent you from eating a variety of foods. For example, eggs and organ meats (such as liver) contain cholesterol, but they also contain many essential vitamins and minerals, as well as protein. Such items can be eaten in moderation, as long as your overall cholesterol intake is not excessive. If you prefer whole milk to skim milk, you can reduce your intake of fats from foods other than milk.

To Avoid Too Much Fat, Saturated Fat, And Cholesterol

• Choose lean meat, fish poultry, dry beans and peas as your protein sources

• Moderate your use of eggs and organ meats (such as liver)

• Limit your intake of butter, cream, hydrogenated margarines, shortenings and coconut oil, and foods made from such products

• Trim excess fat off meats

• Broil, bake or boil rather than fry

• Read labels carefully to determine both amounts and types of fat contained in foods

Eat Foods with Adequate Starch and Fiber

The major sources of energy in the average U.S. diet are carbohydrates and fats. (Proteins and alcohol also supply energy, but to a
lesser extent.) If you limit your fat intake, you should increase your
calories from carbohydrates to supply your body's energy needs.

In trying to reduce your weight to "ideal" levels, carbohydrates have an
advantage over fats: carbohydrates contain less than half the number of
calories per ounce than fats.

Complex carbohydrate foods are better than *simple* carbohydrates in
this regard. Simple carbohydrates — such as sugars — provide calories but
little else in the way of nutrients. Complex carbohydrate foods — such as
beans, peas, nuts, seeds, fruits and vegetables, and whole grain breads,
cereals, and products — contain many essential nutrients in addition to
calories.

Increasing your consumption of certain complex carbohydrates can
also help increase dietary fiber. The average American diet is relatively low
in fiber. Eating more foods high in fiber tends to reduce the symptoms of
chronic constipation, diverticulosis, and some types of "irritable bowel."
There is also concern that low fiber diets might increase the risk of developing cancer of the colon, but whether this is true is not yet known.

To make sure you get enough fiber in your diet, you should eat fruits
and vegetables, whole grain breads and cereals. There is no reason to add
fiber to foods that do not already contain it.

To Eat More Complex Carbohydrates Daily

- Substitute starches for fats and sugars
- Select foods which are good sources of fiber and starch, such as whole
grain breads and cereals, fruits and vegetables, beans, peas, and nuts

Avoid Too Much Sugar

The major health hazard from eating too much sugar is tooth decay
(dental caries). The risk of caries is not simply a matter of how much sugar
you eat. The risk increases the more frequently you eat sugar and sweets,
especially if you eat between meals, and if you eat foods that stick to the
teeth. For example, frequent snacks of sticky candy, or dates, or daylong
use of soft drinks may be more harmful than adding sugar to your morning
cup of coffee — at least as far as your teeth are concerned.

Obviously, there is more to healthy teeth than avoiding sugars. Careful dental hygiene and exposure to adequate amounts of fluoride in the water are especially important.

Contrary to widespread opinion, too much sugar in your diet does not seem to cause diabetes. The most common type of diabetes is seen in obese adults, and avoiding sugar, without correcting the overweight, will not solve the problem. There is also no convincing evidence that sugar causes heart attacks or blood vessel diseases.

Estimates indicate that Americans use on the average more than 130 pounds of sugar and sweeteners a year. This means the risk of tooth decay is increased not only by the sugar in the sugar bowl but by the sugars and syrups in jams, jellies, candies, cookies, soft drinks, cakes, and pies, as well as sugars found in products such as breakfast cereals, catsup, flavored milks, and ice cream. Frequently, the ingredient label will provide a clue to the amount of sugars in a product.

To Avoid Excessive Sugars
• Use less of all sugars, including white sugar, brown sugar, raw sugar, honey, and syrups
• Eat less of foods containing these sugars, such as candy, soft drinks, ice cream, cakes, cookies
• Select fresh fruits or fruits canned without sugar or in light syrup rather than heavy syrup
• Read food labels for clues on sugar content—if the names sucrose, glucose, maltose, dextrose, lactose, fructose, or syrups appear first, then there is a large amount of sugar
• Remember, how often you eat sugar is as important as how much sugar you eat

Avoid Too Much Sodium

Table salt contains sodium and chloride—both are essential elements.

Sodium is also present in many beverages and foods that we eat, especially in certain processed foods, condiments, sauces, pickled foods, salty snacks, and sandwich meats. Baking soda, baking powder, monosodium glutamate (MSG), soft drinks and even many medications (many antacids, for instance) contain sodium.

It is not surprising that adults in the United States take in much more sodium than they need.

The major hazard of excessive sodium is for persons who have high blood pressure. Not everyone is equally susceptible. In the United States, approximately 17% of adults have high blood pressure. Sodium intake is but one of the factors known to affect blood pressure. Obesity, in particular, seems to play a major role.

In populations with low-sodium intakes, high blood pressure is rare. In contrast, in populations with high-sodium intakes, high blood pressure is common. If people with high blood pressure severely restrict their sodium intakes, their blood pressures will *usually* fall – although not always to normal levels.

At present, there is no good way to predict who will develop high blood pressure, though certain groups, such as blacks, have a higher incidence. Low-sodium diets might help some of these people avoid high blood pressure if they could be identified before they develop the condition.

Since most Americans eat more sodium than is needed, consider reducing your sodium intake. Use less table salt. Eat sparingly those foods to which larger amounts of sodium have been added. Remember that up to half of sodium intake may be "hidden," either as part of the naturally occurring food or, more often, as part of a preservative or flavoring agent that has been added.

To Avoid Too Much Sodium
- Learn to enjoy the unsalted flavors of foods
- Cook with only small amounts of added salt
- Add little or no salt to food at the table
- Limit your intake of salty foods, such as potato chips, pretzels, salted nuts and popcorn, condiments (soy sauce, steak sauce, garlic salt), cheese, pickled foods, cured meats
- Read food labels carefully to determine the amount of sodium in processed foods and snack items

If You Drink Alcohol, Do So in Moderation

Alcoholic beverages tend to be high in calories and low in other nutrients. Even moderate drinkers may need to drink less if they wish to achieve ideal weight.

On the other hand, heavy drinkers may lose their appetites for foods containing essential nutrients. Vitamin and mineral deficiencies occur commonly in heavy drinkers – in part, because of poor intake, but also because alcohol alters the absorption and use of some essential nutrients.

Sustained or excessive alcohol consumption by pregnant women has caused birth defects. Pregnant women should limit alcohol intake to 2 ounces or less on any single day.

Heavy drinking may also cause a variety of serious conditions, such as cirrhosis of the liver and some neurological disorders. Cancer of the throat and neck is much more common in people who drink and smoke than in people who don't.

One or two drinks daily appear to cause no harm to adults. If you drink you should do so in moderation.

NOTE: These recommendations are intended only for populations with food habits similar to people in the United States.
U.S. Department of Agriculture
U.S. Department of Health and Human Services
Home and Garden Bulletin No. 232
Previously issued as an unnumbered publication.

REFERENCES

1. *Webster's New World Dictionary, College Edition.*Cleveland, The World Publishing Company, 1962, p 322.

2. *Webster's New World Dictionary, College Edition.* Cleveland, The World Publishing Company, 1962, p 3.

3. Olson RE: Clinical nutrition, an interface between human ecology and internal medicine. *Nutr Rev* 36:161, 1978.

4. Mann GV: The influence of obesity in health. *N Engl J Med* 291:178; 226, 1974.

5. Select Committee on Nutritional and Human Needs, US Senate: (Revised) *Dietary Goals for the United States.* Washington, US Government Printing Office, 1978.

6. Harper AE: Dietary goals – a skeptical view. *Am J Clin Nutr* 31:310, 1978.

7. Committee of Principal Investigators: A cooperative trial in the primary prevention of ischaemic heart disease using clofibrate. *Br Heart J* 40:1069, 1978.

8. Pearce ML, Dayton S: Incidence of cancer in men on a diet high in polyunsaturated fat. *Lancet* 1:464, 1971.

9. Broad WJ: Nutrition's battle of the Potomac. *Nutr Today* 14(4):6–13, 1979.

10. Hegsted DM: Dietary goals – a progressive view. *Am J Clin Nutr* 31:1504, 1978.

11. National Dairy Council: Cholesterol Metabolism. *Dairy Council Digest* 50(6):31–35. 1979.

12. Mann GV: Diet-heart: end of an era. *N Engl J Med* 297:644, 1977.

2 Can We Design an Optimal Diet for the United States?

Robert E. Olson, MD, PhD

At the present time, there is unprecedented interest in the subject of nutrition in the country by the people, by consumer advocate groups, by health food advocates, by voluntary health agencies like the American Heart Association and the American Cancer Society, and by the US Government through the National Institutes of Health and various Congressional committees. All are advising the American public what to do about diet to prevent chronic disease. The question is: are we ready? Is the data base underlying such recommendations firm?

The Food and Nutrition Board of the National Academy of Sciences was founded in 1941 to make recommendations to a country at war regarding nutritional allowances that would maintain a high level of health and productivity in our population. In the interval since 1941, the Food and Nutrition Board has deliberated nine times with regard to essential nutrients, making recommendations for daily intake that will provide "levels of intake of essential nutrients which in their judgment and on the basis of available scientific knowledge will be adequate to meet the known nutritional needs of practically all healthy persons."[1] Of the 45 known chemicals required for normal nutrition in human beings, the Food and

Nutrition Board has gradually increased the number of nutrients for which Recommended Dietary Allowances (RDAs) were made, from 8 in 1943 to 18 in 1978. This reflects the evolutionary nature of the Board's deliberations with regard to an expanding data base. The question now is, can the Board go beyond the RDAs in recommending changes in the ratio of macronutrients such as fat and carbohydrate or in the intake of vitamins and minerals beyond the basic requirements?

The Dietary Goals for the United States, a document published by the Senate Select Committee on Nutrition and Human Needs, has been the center of intense controversy since it was issued in early 1977.[2] There have been stands taken for and against. Without taking a formal stand on the value of the Committee's report at this time, let me say in principle that I believe in selective dietary goals beyond those implicit in the RDAs. I doubt that any single dietary recommendation, however, will be appropriate for all segments of our population, ie, infants, children, young men, pregnant and lactating women, nonpregnant women before menopause, women after menopause, and men and women beyond age 70. The frontier in public health and nutrition is moving and we must be prepared to both make and criticize recommendations that are made to secure optimal diets for given segments of our population, as our data base expands. The following criteria appear useful to me in developing a critique for judging such recommendations.

1. Epidemiologic studies are not, of themselves, sufficient evidence to assume cause-and-effect relationships between associated health variables. For example, when Robert Koch discovered the tubercle bacillus, the general view of epidemiologists of his time was that tuberculosis was a disease of malnutrition. He had to demonstrate in the laboratory by application of his four postulates that the tubercle bacillus was, in fact, the agent of the disease. On the other hand, when Joseph Goldberger began to investigate pellagra in the southern United States, the prevailing view, based on the epidemiology available at the time, was that pellagra was a disease of infection. By careful epidemiologic and clinical studies, Goldberger showed that it was a disease of malnutrition.

2. In diseases of multiple etiology in which genetic factors are apparent, it is necessary to understand the extent to which dietary intervention can be successful under the best conditions.

3. Clinical intervention trials using the recommended dietary regimen in the population at risk should be positive before public health education is contemplated. In the case of scurvy, diet intervention with citrus fruits cured the disease; the lime supplements to the diet of healthy sailors prevented its appearance. In the case of pellagra, feeding either animal protein or nicotinic acid prevented and/or cured the disease. It would seem important to demand similar evidence of the efficacy of diet change in given chronic diseases before recommending sweeping changes in the US diet.

4. Strong support from the medical and paramedical professions for a contemplated dietary change to control disease should be secured before initiating a given public health nutrition program.

The debate about the need for dietary change in the United States to reduce chronic degenerative disease will no doubt continue for years. Some comfort is provided by the fact that the coronary disease rate in this country has been decreasing since 1960. Diet and other aspects of lifestyle have also been changing spontaneously, and this dynamic system requires more study to determine the relevant variables. We can feel secure in recommending to the public weight control, improved physical fitness, cessation of cigarette smoking, and control of hypertension and diabetes. Beyond that, much still needs to be learned.

REFERENCES

1. Committee on Dietary Allowances, Food and Nutrition Board: *Recommended Dietary Allowances*, ed 9. Washington, DC, National Academy of Sciences, 1980.
2. Select Committee on Nutritional and Human Needs, US Senate: *Dietary Goals for the United States*, ed 2. Washington, DC, US Government Printing Office, 1977.

SUGGESTED READINGS

Ahrens EH: The management of hyperlipidemias: whether, rather than how. *Ann Intern Med* 85:87–93 1976.
Dietary Goals for the United States: A Commentary. Council for Agricultural Science and Technology, Washington, US Government Printing Office, 1977.
Truswell AS: Diet and plasma lipids — a reappraisal. *Am J Clin Nutr* 311:977–989 1978.

3 Human Milk Versus Proprietary Milk in the Newborn

Ophilia James, MD

Until recently it was felt that human milk and formula based on cow's milk were much the same biochemically and nutritionally. In fact, the constituents of cow's milk and human milk are dissimilar in almost all respects, with the exception of water and lactose, and even these are quantitatively different.

Modification has made cow's milk less inappropriate for the human infant. However, the history of formula production has been a series of errors, particularly for the premature infant. Adding substances in formula like emulsifiers, thickening agents, pH adjusters, antioxidants, carrageenan, and hydroxypropyl starch introduces further unknown substances that are not found in the original product.

Apprehension began 15 years ago with widespread acceptance of bottle-feeding, with two separate groups: pediatric nutritionists in tropical countries, worried by the increase in diarrhea and marasmus, and women's groups in industrialized countries. Recently, scientific support for breast-feeding has emerged from a range of disciplines including neonatologists, allergists, and immunologists.

Table 3-1 shows the composition of milks obtained from various species and the growth rates of their offspring. It is obvious that the nutrient density is highest in milk produced by the fastest-growing species. This illustrates the assumption that breast milk alone is specifically composed for the human newborn with regard to its nutrient density in relation to the growth rate of the human infant.

Table 3-1
Composition of Milks Obtained from Different Mammals
and the Growth Rate of Their Offspring

Species	Days Required to Double Birth Weight	Content of Milk (%)			
		Fat	Protein	Lactose	Ash
Man	180	3.8	0.9	7.0	0.2
Horse	60	1.9	2.5	6.2	0.5
Cow	47	3.7	3.4	4.8	0.7
Reindeer	30	16.9	11.5	2.8	
Goat	19	4.5	2.9	4.1	0.8
Sheep	10	7.4	5.5	4.8	1.0
Rat	6	15.0	12.0	3.0	2.0

From Hambraeus.[1] Reprinted with permission.

In human milk, fat provides about 50% of the calories, lactose is the major carbohydrate, and the vitamin and mineral content is lower than in cow's milk formula. Lactose has been shown to increase iron absorption in the gut. McMillian et al[2] have shown that infants fed solely on human milk will maintain a positive iron balance, in contrast to formula-fed infants.

Whey proteins represent more than 70% of the total protein in breast milk, but only 20% of the total cow's milk protein. Whey proteins are the non-curd-forming proteins. There is a further difference in the composition of whey proteins in the two milks: whereas β-lactoglobulin is the dominating cow's milk whey protein, it is absent in human milk. β lactoglobulin is the commonest food allergen in infancy. About 1% of bottle-fed infants can be found to be affected in industrialized countries.[3] Alpha lactalbumin is the major whey protein in human milk. Lactoferrin is the iron-binding protein and represents the other dominating whey protein component in breast milk; it occurs in very small amounts in cow's milk. Since bacteria require iron for growth, lactoferrin inhibits the growth of several pathogens. It has been said to contribute to a large extent to the marked resistance against infectious gastroenteritis caused by *Escherichia coli*.

The other two important whey proteins are secretory IgA and lysozyme. Secretory IgA has been shown to be present in the intestine of breast-fed infants and participates in the defense mechanism by binding viruses and bacteria.[4,5] Lysozyme has an indirect bacterial effect by potentiating the activity of immune antibodies. Casein, the other milk protein, is found in much larger amounts in cow's milk. It is the curd-forming protein. There are important physiochemical differences in the composition of casein in the two milks. Additionally, antistaphylococcal factor, complement components, and macrophages are other important components of human milk absent in cow's milk. The macrophages have been presumed to originate from maternal blood monocytes that migrate to the mammary gland in the last months of pregnancy.

Now that we have looked at the differences in composition of cow's milk formula and human milk, let us look at their implications in disease states.

Diarrhea

Colonization of the neonatal gut occurs during the first few days of life. The formula-fed infant's gut flora is similar to that of an older child by the end of the first week of life, ie, there is colonization with *E coli*, bacteroides, *Clostridia,* and a few *Lactobacilli.* By contrast, in the breast-fed infant, by the end of the first 3 to 4 days of life a stable, rich microflora develops, 99% of which is *Lactobacillus bifidus.*[5] This contributes to the low pH of breast-milk stools. There is consequently a paucity of putrefactive bacteria. The frequency of diarrheal deaths at the turn of the century was six times greater in British infants fed cow's milk, than those fed human milk. Half a century later, it was discovered that the incidence of enteric and respiratory infections and infant morbidity and mortality rates was substantially lower in breast-fed infants.

Gastrointestinal Allergies

During the immediate postpartum period, particularly in premature and small-for-gestational-age infants, as a result of delay in maturation of the mucosal barrier, newborn infants are particularly susceptible to pathologic penetration by harmful intraluminal substances, leading to increased susceptibility to infection, potential for hypersensitivity reactions, and potential for the formation of immune complexes. Breast milk prevents these by forming a mucosal barrier and facilitating intestinal maturation.[5]

It appears (Table 3-2) that virtually every deficiency or delay in maturation of host defenses is countered by a factor in breast milk. Widdowson[6] has shown that the gastrointestinal epithelium proliferates and matures more rapidly in experimental animals given maternal milk than in those given isocaloric substitute formula. Others have shown that brush-border enzymes are enhanced by colostrum.

24

Table 3-2
Immature Newborn Intestinal Host Defenses vs Passive Protective Factors in Human Milk

Immature Intestinal Host Defenses	Human Milk Factors
Gastric barrier	Acidification properties
Absence of indigenous flora	of milk
	Bifidus factor
	Antistaphylococcal factor
	Lysozyme
Secretory IgA deficiency	Milk antibodies (predominantly secretory IgA)
	(?) Adjuvant effect on local immune system
Enhanced antigen/bacterial permeability	Intestinal "Epidermal" maturation factor
Enhanced bacterial adherence	(?) Glycoprotein inhibitors of bacterial adherence

From Walker.[5] Reprinted with permission.

The increased permeability of the neonatal gut to macromolecules leads to absorption of antigenic quantities of proteins.[5] Although the mechanisms of gastrointestinal allergies are not completely understood, it would appear that the intestinal transport of macromolecules is a necessary initial step. During the period of increased neonatal gut permeability, susceptible individuals may become sensitized to ingested protein and, with later re-exposure to minute but sufficient quantities of allergens, develop allergic symptoms.

An altered gut epithelium, as after an episode of gastroenteritis, may predispose susceptible infants to sensitizing qualities of allergens; or an underdeveloped secretory immune system may also allow for uptake of critical amounts of sensitizing proteins.

The following clinical conditions in newborns are possibly associated with intestinal host defenses[5] (Reprinted with permission):

Immediate Disease States
   Necrotizing enterocolitis
   Gastrointestinal allergy
   Sudden infant death syndrome
   Dermatitis enteropathica
Delayed Disease States
   Inflammatory bowel disease
   Chronic active hepatitis
   Nephritis
   Autoimmune diseases

Delayed Disease States

The pathogenesis of inflammatory bowel disease is unclear. One of the current hypotheses is that bacterial antigens taken up from the intestine lead to a local hypersensitivity reaction. This in turn causes mucosal ulceration and granulomatous reaction. To support this hypothesis, antibodies cytotoxic to normal colonic cell suspensions have been reported in sera of patients with inflammatory bowel disease. In recent clinical reports, the suggestion has been made that milk antigens absorbed during infancy may predispose to complex diseases such as chronic active hepatitis and nephritis.

Necrotizing Enterocolitis

This disease illustrates the association between altered host defenses and the pathogenesis of clinical disease. The condition is in all likelihood directly related to defective gut mechanisms (gut injury) that retain bacteria on the surface of the small intestine.

Table 3-3 shows precipitating factors in necrotizing enterocolitis (NEC) pathogenesis. The condition usually progresses rapidly with signs of vomiting, abdominal distension, obstruction and, finally, if severe enough, perforation. X-ray findings are diagnostic, showing air pockets within the distal small intestinal lumen. Despite extensive epidemiologic research no specific bacterial species has been implicated in this condition. In fact, Virnig and Reynolds[8] suggest that organisms involved in NEC are normal bowel flora that enter the peritoneum and bloodstream through an altered gut mucosa. Barlow et al[9] have direct evidence that macrophages present in breast milk may provide passive protection against bacterial penetration.

Table 3-3
Pathogenesis of NEC — Precipitating Factors

1. Infection	4. Oral feedings
2. Endotoxin	5. Mucosal injury
3. Mucosal ischemia	6. Altered host defense

From Lake and Walker.[7] Reprinted with permission

The three essential components in the pathogenesis of NEC[10] are:
Injury to the intestinal mucosa
Intestinal microflora
Availability of metabolic substrate (feedings)
Figure 3-1 summarizes the proposed mechanisms for development of NEC. By virtue of the protective effects of human milk, breast-fed infants very rarely, if ever, develop NEC.

26

Other aspects of breast milk vs formula include:

1. Maternal-infant bonding. The positive effect of breast-feeding on maternal-infant relationship and bonding has been recently emphasized.[3,11,12] The formation of intense attachment has been shown to be related to physical contact leading to mutually reinforcing reflex behavior occurring most readily during a sensitive period, ie, during the first 24 hours of life, especially with biologic breast-feeding.

2. Breast-feeding protects against overfeeding and obesity. During breast-feeding, the associated changes in taste and texture of milk (higher fat content toward the end of the feeding episode) may be factors in the infant's decrease in appetite and suckling, and termination of the nursing episode.

3. Child spacing. Estimates indicate that in the world today, lactation amenorrhea has a larger statistical effect on protection for a few years than currently available technologic contraceptive programs.[4]

4. Economics. Breast-feeding conserves resources in the ingredients

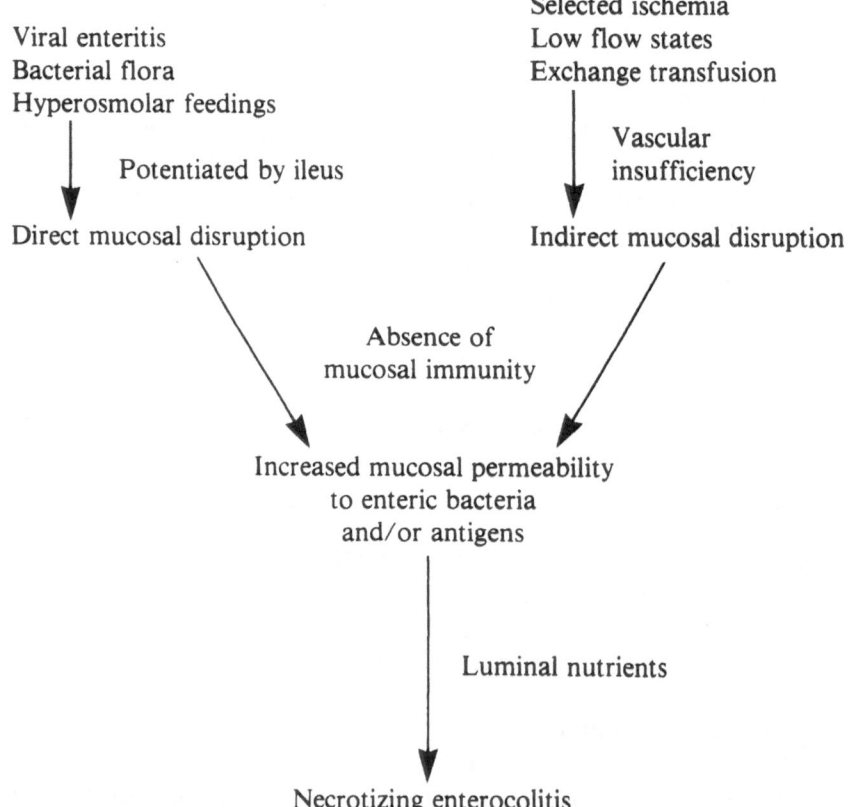

Figure 3-1 Proposed mechanisms for the development of NEC. From Lake and Walker.[7] Reprinted with permission.

Table 3-4
Advisable Intakes of Growing Premature Infants and Composition of Feeding

	Advisable Intakes*		Composition			
	800 to 1200 gm 26 to 29 weeks	1200 to 1800 gm 29 to 32 weeks	Human Milk	Similac, Enfamil, SMA	Enfamil Premature	Similac 24 LBW
Protein (gm)	3.1	2.7	1.5	2.2	3.0	2.7
Sodium (mEq)	2.7	2.3	0.8	1.0-2.5	1.7	2.0
Chloride (mEq)	2.4	2.0	1.7	1.5-3.6	2.4	3.0
Potassium (mEq)	1.9	1.8	1.2	2.1-4.2	2.8	3.2
Calcium (mg)	160	140	43	66-90	117	90
Phosphorus (mg)	108	95	20	49-68	58	70
Magnesium (mg)	7.5	6.5	5	6-8	10	10

*Values per 100 kcal.
From E.E. Ziegler, personal communication, 1980.

28

used, in the material for canning, and in the money consumed for production and distribution. This has a very significant bearing on resource-poor developing nations.

At the family level the cost of breast milk versus bottle has been much discussed. In developing countries, to formula-feed a baby would take 20% to 50% of the family income. Overall, bottle-feeding has been estimated to be 2 to 3 times more expensive than breast-feeding. Breast-feeding is a prophylactic against marasmus in disadvantaged countries and against obesity in more affluent circumstances.

Breast Milk and the Premature Infant

It appears that breast milk alone is not ideal for the premature infant. Fomon and Ziegler[13,14] have shown that breast milk is inadequate in its protein and mineral content (particularly sodium), for the premature infant; prematures require a higher protein-energy and mineral-energy ratio than is present in breast milk.

REFERENCES

1. Hambraeus L: Proprietary milk versus human milk in infant feeding. A critical appraisal from the nutritional point of view. *Pediatr Clin North Am* 24:17–36, 1977.
2. McMillian JA, Landaw SA, Oski FA: Iron sufficiency in breast fed infants and the availability of iron from human milk. *Pediatrics* 58:686–691, 1976.
3. Goldman AS: Sensitivity to cow milk. *Proceedings of XIII Swedish Nutrition Foundation Symposium on Food and Immunology*, Stockholm, Swedish Nutrition Foundation, 1977 p 99.
4. Goldman AS: Immunologic factors and leukocytes in human milk. *Mead Johnson Symp Perinat Dev Med* 11:49–53, 1977.
5. Walker WA: Development of intestinal host defense mechanisms and the passive protective role of human milk. *Mead Johnson Symp Perinat Dev Med* 11:39–48, 1977.
6. Widdowson EM: Changes in the body and its organs during lactation: nutritional implications, in Elliott K, Fitzsimons DW (eds): *Breast-Feeding and the Mother*. Elsevier, Netherlands, Mouton Publishers, 1976, pp 103–118.
7. Lake AM, Walker WA: Neonatal necrotizing enteroclitis: A disease of altered host defense. *Clin Gastroenterol* 6(2): 463–480, 1977.
8. Virnig NL, Reynolds JW: Epidemiological aspects of neonatal necrotizing enterocolitis. *Am J Dis Child* 128:186, 1974.
9. Barlow B, Santulli TV, Heird WC, et al: An experimental study of acute necrotizing enterocolitis – the importance of breast milk. *J Pediatr Surg* 9:587, 1974.
10. Santulli TV, Schullinger JN, Heird WC, et al: Acute necrotizing enterocolitis in infancy: a review of 64 cases. *Pediatrics* 55(3):376–87, 1975.
11. Klaus MH, Kennell JH, Plum N et al: Human maternal behavior at the first contact with her young. *Pediatrics* 46:187–192, 1970.
12. Klaus MH, Kennell JH: Human maternal and paternal behavior, in Klaus

MH, Kennell JH (eds): *Maternal Infant Bonding.* St. Louis, CV Mosby Co, 1976, pp 38–98.

13. Fomon SJ, Zeigler EE: Milk of the premature infant's mother: interpretation of data. *J Pediatr* 93:164, 1978.

14. Fomon SJ, Ziegler EE, Vasquez HD: Human milk and the small premature infant. *Am J Dis Child* 131:463, 1977.

4 Does Human Milk Intrinsically Help Protect Newborns from Infection?

Neal S. LeLeiko, MD, PhD

The purpose of this presentation is to discuss the contents of human milk from the standpoint of specific agents that might serve to protect the newborn infant from infectious disease. There are many factors in human milk for which an immunologic role has been proposed. It is necessary to assess the functions of these different factors as well as to determine whether any of these factors might be expected to survive in the infant's digestive tract. Finally, assuming that an immunologically active agent is capable of performing its action in the newborn, it is necessary to look at the evidence as to whether an actual significant immune effect is served. This latter task can be approached only through a review of the published epidemiologic studies on breast-feeding.

Possible Host Resistance Factors

The contents of human milk that might be expected to have anti-infection properties are:
Antibodies

Cells
Growth factor for *Lactobacillus bifidus*
Antistaphylococcal factor
Complement (C_3, C_4)
Lysozyme
Lactoperoxidase
Lactoferrin
Other binding proteins
Antiviral factors

Antibodies All classes of immunoglobulins (or antibodies) are found in human milk. Colostrum, which has the highest concentration of immunoglobulins, has an exceptionally high concentration of immunoglobulin A (IgA). The IgA is in the form of secretory IgA. Selner et al[1] in a study of salivary immunoglobulins in the neonatal period, attempted to detect secretory IgA at different ages. At 10 days of age, less than 10% of the neonates studied had detectable secretory IgA in their saliva. The percentage did not reach 90% until almost 4 weeks of age. Thus, from a teleologic viewpoint we can appreciate that the high level of secretory IgA present in breast milk, especially in colostrum and early milk, may not be accidental.

There is no question that a significant quantity of antibodies is present in human milk. It is interesting to note that these antibodies have been shown to be more resistant to pepsin and acid digestion than serum antibodies.[2] Shim et al[3] have shown that colostral IgA is intrinsically resistant to tryptic digestion, and indeed others[4] have demonstrated a specific trypsin inhibitor in colostrum during the first five days of life.

Many authors have demonstrated the presence of specific antibodies in infant stool, thus verifying that these antibodies, at least, survive through passage in the infant intestinal tract. Furthermore, these coproantibodies have been found to correlate with maternal serum antibody levels and are absent from similar bottle-fed infants.

Thus, there seems to be ample support for the statement that the antibodies survive infant digestion. We must still inquire whether they function and, if so, how?

Elegant mechanisms of macromolecular absorption by neonatal mammalian intestine have been put forth.[5] A specific selective mechanism for the transport of maternal gamma globulins has also been presumed to be present in many mammals. There is, however, no evidence that this system has any significance in the human intestine. More likely, the action of antibodies in human milk is limited to the alimentary tract of the neonate. It appears as though secretory IgA binds antigen in the lumen of the intestine before the antigen can be absorbed. The binding would be expected to have several results. It might intrinsically "deactivate" the antigen. More likely, the binding results in the formation of large aggregates of antibody and antigen, and thus decreases the efficiency of absorption of the antigen. This decreased absorptive capacity means that the antigen will have increased exposure to other environmental agents present in the intestine. These would include digestive enzymes as well as other factors.

Cells There are between 2000 and 4000 cells per ml in colostrum. Approximately 80% to 90% are large, ameboid, highly phagocytic macrophages. Approximately 10% are lymphocytes. Of the lymphocytes about 50% are T cells and 30% are B cells; the rest are not readily identifiable. The T cell population appears to be a specific subpopulation of cells and not a cross-section of blood lymphocytes.

There is some evidence to suggest that the T cells may transport important mediator molecules such as transfer factor.[6,7] It has been reported that PPD-positive mothers who breast fed were likely to have infants who were also PPD-positive.[6,7] That this observed effect is the result of immunity transferred through breast milk is not certain, and therefore this important result cannot be considered conclusive.

The actual role of the lymphocytes is uncertain. The pH of the gastric secretions of the newborn is relatively high because of diminished gastric secretion of HCl. Therefore, it is likely that leukocytes may enter the small intestine. Pitt[8] showed in a rat model that a *Klebsiella*-induced necrotizing enterocolitis could be prevented by feeding rat colostral macrophages.

There is evidence that the macrophage may actually be serving as an immunoglobulin transport vehicle and that, as such, it is capable of delayed release of immunoglobulins over several days. It has been suggested that in vitro differentiation of milk lymphocytes into IgA-secreting plasma cells may be a significant factor in the large amount of IgA theoretically utilized by the infant.[9].

Growth factor for *Lactobacillus bifidus* The intestine of breast-fed newborns is quickly colonized by *Lacotobacillus bifidus*, whereas other infants develop a mixed bacterial flora. The lactobacillus produces acetic acid and lactic acid, which results in a decreased stool pH. In vitro this acidic environment inhibits the growth of such potential pathogens as *Escherichia coli, Shigella,* and certain yeasts.

The bifidus factor (methyl-N-acetyl d-glucosamine) is a specific growth factor that promotes the growth of *L bifidus.* Thus the change in flora is the result of two effects, ie, inhibition of other bacteria by the metabolic products of *L bifidus,* as well as the promotion of the growth of the lactobacillus by a specific factor. Although the change in the flora is not debatable, there are many who question the significance of the changed flora with regard to the actual incidence of infectious disease.

Antistaphylococcal factor In the preantibiotic era it was observed that milk given parenterally to laboratory animals seemed to have a specific therapeutic effect on the animals who had been subjected to a standard in-oculum of staphylococci. The factor responsible appears to be a C18:2 fatty acid. The significance of this factor in humans is completely obscure.

Complement (C_3, C_4) The presence of C_3 and C_4 in human milk has been somewhat of a mystery. Together these factors participate in the facilitation of bacterial killing. The initiating components of the classic pathway of complement activation are, however, not present in human milk; therefore, until recently there had been little reason to suspect the C_3 and C_4 of breast milk to have any significant immunologic role. Studies[10] have now demonstrated the presence of C_3 proactivator in breast milk. This allows for activation of the complement system via the alternative pathway. Thus C_3 and C_4 may indeed be immunologically active components of breast milk.

Lysozyme This is an enzyme that attacks bacterial cell walls. There is a very high concentration of lysozyme in human milk, over 300 times that in cow's milk. The enzyme is stable at acid pH and therefore remains active during infant digestion. It has been assayed in infant stools and found to be present in significantly greater amounts in the stools of breast-fed infants than in the stools of bottle-fed infants. It is possible that its effect is a synergistic one, ie, by attacking bacteria present in the intestinal lumen that have already been acted on by other factors.

Lactoperoxidase This enzyme system is effective in the killing of streptococci in vitro. There is no evidence to suggest that it has any significant in vivo effect on infective organisms.

Lactoferrin This is an iron-binding protein present in external secretions. The concentration of this protein is higher in milk than in any other body fluid. The protein has an extremely high affinity for iron, even greater than that for transferrin. It is postulated that since many pathogenic bacteria seem to require significant amounts of iron for multiplication, the lactoferrin may inhibit bacterial growth by removing the iron from the environment of the bacteria. Once deprived of this essential nutrient the bacteria could not continue to multiply. We can only speculate at this time on the immune function.

Other binding proteins There are present in human milk binding proteins for folic acid and vitamin B_{12}. It has been suggested that these proteins might function to deprive growing bacteria of essential nutrients in a manner analogous to that postulated for lactoferrin. The role of such binding proteins remains unknown.

Antiviral factors Breast milk contains a number of such factors, including interferon and various fatty acids. Many of these agents have antiviral actions; some of these are quite nonspecific. It is unclear whether these factors are specific to human milk. Additionally, a possible anti-infective role remains to be elaborated.

Epidemiologic Considerations

The question remains whether the breast-fed infant derives an intrinsic immunologic advantage from the ingestion of breast milk. To determine this it is necessary to have a controlled prospective study in which all environmental factors other than mode of feeding have been matched. It is, however, extremely difficult if not impossible to conduct such a study, and no such study has been made. There are a number of retrospective epidemiologic investigations that have attempted to provide an answer to this question. When examined as a whole, these provide compelling evidence that breast-fed infants are sick less often and less severely than infants who are bottle-fed.

A classic study by Robinson[11] showed that wholly bottle-fed infants had greater morbidity rates for gastroenteritis, respiratory infections, and otitis media. Furthermore, the infections tended to be longer and to result in a greater mortality among partially and wholly bottle-fed infants. Infants who were partially breast-fed seemed to do better than those who were wholly bottle-fed, but not as well as those wholly breast-fed. No difference was demonstrated among social classes. (Table 4-1.)

Table 4-1
Morbidity and Case Mortality according to Type of Feeding

	Morbidity per 1000	Case Mortality (%)
Breast-fed	223.4	4.6
Partially breast-fed	464.7	5.5
Bottle-fed	573.7	10.0

From Robinson.[11] Reprinted with permission.

In Sweden, Sydow and Faxen[12] examined a homogeneous population in a children's home. Infants were divided into a group that received a standard formula, and a group that received human milk (pooled) via bottle. In this very limited study there were fewer episodes of increased fever in the human-milk–fed group. This study is interesting because conditions were identical for both groups. Unfortunately, there is no practical way to repeat this experiment with an adequate number of subjects and for a sufficiently long period to answer the question at hand. Nonetheless, it serves as a model for the examination of the effect of human milk, but only in terms of pooled breast milk. The question of the effect of one mother's milk would still be unanswered.

Mellander et al[13] found that the incidence of acute infection, including otitis media, febrile upper respiratory tract infection, and acute diarrhea, was significantly decreased in breast-fed infants aged 3 months to 1 year. Larsen and Homer[14] reviewed their experience with patients in a homogeneous middle-class population suffering from acute diarrhea and requiring hospitalization. Of 35 infants who were admitted to their hospital, who had been followed since birth, only one was being breast-fed at the time of admission. This is despite an estimated overall breast-fed population varying between 39% during the first month of life and 17% at 6 months.

Cunningham[15] reviewed the records of children under 1 year of age at an upstate New York medical center and found that there were significantly fewer episodes of otitis media, acute lower respiratory illness, and significant vomiting and diarrhea among infants who were being breast-fed. Overall, he found significantly more hospital admissions among bottle-fed infants than among breast-fed infants. The advantage for breast-fed infants seemed to remain for the entire first year of life. (Table 4-2)

Table 4-2
**Episodes of Illness per 1000 Patient Weeks Divided by
Method of Feeding**

	Breast-Fed	Artificially Fed
Otitis media	3.4	6.3
Acute lower respiratory infection	0.34	5.5
Vomiting or diarrhea	2.0	4.9
Admissions to hospital	0.34	2.9
Total episodes of illness	5.8	16.8

From Cunningham AS: Morbidity in breast-fed and artificially fed infants. *J Pediatr* 90: 726, 1977. Reprinted with permission.

Conclusions

We can thus draw the following conclusions: 1) There are a number of factors present in human milk that could have an immunologic role. 2) These host resistance factors are capable of surviving in the newborn's intestinal tract. 3) There is sound theoretical reasoning as well as good evidence that many of these factors function in the newborn. 4) There is epidemiologic evidence to support the contention that these host resistance factors provide an intrinsic immunologic advantage to the breast-fed baby.

REFERENCES

1. Selner JC, Merrill DA, Claman HN: Salivary immunoglobulin and albumin: development during the neonatal period. *J Pediatr* 72:685, 1968.

2. Kenny JF, Boesman MI, Michaels RH: Bacterial and viral coproantibodies in breast-fed infants. *Pediatrics* 39:202, 1967.

3. Shim BS, Kang YS, Kim WJ, et al: Self-protective activity of colostral IgA against tryptic digestion. *Nature* 222:787, 1969.

4. Laskowski M, Laskowski M: Crystalline trypsin inhibitor from colostrum. *J Biol Chem* 190:563, 1951.

5. Walker WA, Isselbacher K: Uptake and transport of macromolecules by the intestine: possible role in clinical disorders. *Gastroenterology* 67:531, 1974.

6. Mohr JA: Lymphocyte sensitization passed to the child from the mother. *Lancet* 1:688, 1972.

7. Mohr JA: The possible induction and/or acquisition of cellular hypersensitivity associated with ingestion of colostrum. *J Pediatr* 82:1062, 1972.

8. Pitt J: Passive transfer of milk phagocytes — mechanisms of protection in necrotizing enterocolitis in Moore TD (ed): *Necrotizing Enterocolitis in the Newborn Infant, Sixty-eighth Ross Conference on Pediatric Research,* Columbus, Ohio, Ross Laboratories, 1975, p 52.

9. Murillo GJ, Goldman AS: The cells of human colostrum II. Synthesis of IgA and B1c. *Pediatr Res* 4:71, 1970.

10. Ballow M, Fang F, Good RA, et al: Developmental aspects of complement components and C^3 proactivator (properdin factor B) in human colostrum. *Clin Exp Immunol* 18:257, 1974.

11. Robinson M: Infant morbidity and mortality. A study of 3266 infants. *Lancet* 1:788, 1951.

12. Sydow GV, Faxen N: Breast or cow's milk as infant food: discussion on the methods of comparison. *Acta Paediatr Scand* 43:362, 1974.

13. Mellander O, Vahlquist D, Mellbin T: Breast feeding and artificial feeding. A clinical, serological and biochemical study in 402 infants with a survey of the literature. The Norrbotten Study. *Acta Paediatr Scand [Suppl]* 48:(116):1, 1959.

14. Larsen SA Jr, Homer DR: Relation of breast versus bottle feeding to hospitalization for gastroenteritis in a middle-class U.S. population. *J Pediatr* 92:417, 1978.

15. Cunningham AS: Morbidity in breast-fed and artificially fed infants. *J Pediatr* 90:726, 1977.

5 Psychosocial Aspects of Breast-Feeding

Kathleen J. Motil, MD, PhD

For many years, bottle-feeding has been the primary method of nurturing infants. Social pressures and public health sanctions have continued to foster this trend. Recent evidence suggests, however, that there are distinct advantages to breast-feeding when compared to bottle-feeding.[1] More specifically, the biochemical and immunologic constituents of human milk confer a uniqueness and species-specificity not achieved in commercial milk preparations or cow's milk.[2] Biochemical uniqueness is demonstrated by difference in amino acid levels, such as elevated taurine and cystine and lowered tyrosine and phenylalanine concentrations,[3,4] the absence of sensitizing proteins such as β-lactoglobulin, and a greater proportion of proteins of high biologic value in the whey fraction of human milk.[5] Not only are protein constituents unique, but lipid fractions also differ from other mammalian milks. Human milk contains greater amounts of 2-monoglycerides, thereby enhancing fat absorption.[6] Human milk also contains a lipase that preferentially liberates fatty acids from the 1- and 3-positions in order to facilitate absorption.[7] Finally, many biochemical constituents of human milk have interdependent interactions. For example, both human and cow's milks contain similar iron and zinc concentrations; however, absorption of both minerals is more effective in human milk.[8,9] In addition to these biochemical features, human milk contains many immunologic factors that provide protection against illness in the young infant.[10,11] Cellular components, particularly the lymphocytes and macrophages, perform essential functions related to bacterial killing and cell-mediated immunity.[12] There are a host of specific antibodies, such as antistaphylococcal antibodies, the lactobacillis factor, and secretory IgA, that promote resistance to infections in the young infant. All of these features in human milk impart a distinct advantage to the human organism compared to that of cow's milk or commercial preparations.

In addition to these biochemical and immunologic factors, there are other aspects of breast-feeding infrequently acknowledged and certainly not well-studied. These are the psychosocial aspects of breast-feeding; they will provide the topic for consideration in this chapter. The term psychosocial has broad implications and encompasses a range of topics beyond the scope of this chapter. For our purposes here, the focus of information will center on three areas of interest: 1) maternal-infant bonding, 2) lactational infertility, and 3) child development.

The material that provides insight into the psychosocial aspects of breast-feeding relies heavily on behavioral studies in both animals and humans. It is important to note that behavioral studies in humans are much more difficult to design and carry out, compared to general behavioral studies in animals, as well as studies that ask basic physiologic and biochemical questions. In addition, human behavioral studies are laden with biases that are difficult either to remove or to control. For example, mothers who breast-feed have a unique set of attitudes concerning child-rearing practices. These attitudes constitute a bias that cannot be duplicated in a control set of mothers. Finally, many of the previously published reports are retrospective studies that have failed to examine or control interactions among multiple environmental factors. Therefore, behavioral studies related to breast-feeding must be interpreted with caution.

Maternal-Infant Bonding

From the teleologic point of view, breast-feeding has evolved to meet the nutritional and immunologic needs of the newborn infant. Lactation also provides the natural opportunity for early bonding between the mother and infant. Bonding is an essential element in the mother-child relationship, since this attachment is critical for both the physical survival and the psychologic adjustment of the infant.[13] Because of the complexity of human behavior, however, the nature of this interaction has been characterized in animal models.[14]

The importance of bonding is demonstrated by observations from behavioral studies in goats.[15] In these studies, female goats were divided into two groups: The experimental group consisted of newly delivered mothers, separated from their young immediately after parturition, while the control group of mothers was allowed normal contact with its kids. After one hour, the kids from the experimental group were returned to their mothers. The mother-kid interactions from both groups were observed repeatedly during 15-minute intervals. In the control group of intact mother-kid pairs, the young displayed continuous feeding behavior in all cases. In contrast, however, the mothers in the early separation group ignored their young and continued eating. Moreover, this pattern of indifferent behavior by the mothers did not resolve with increasing maternal-young contact. Even after two months, the separated mothers nursed other kids as often as their own, while mothers from the intact group refused to nurse foreign kids and often butted them away.

In animals, lactation starts immediately after birth and is the natural means by which bonding is established. Bonding thereby provides the means to achieve appropriate caretaking of the young by the mother. The influence of lactation on maternal caretaking behavior has been described in studies using mice as the animal model.[16] These studies consisted of newly delivered mice that were divided into two groups: the test group of mothers was unable to lactate because their nipples had been surgically removed prior to parturition, while the control group consisted of mothers who received a sham operation. Mothers from each group were placed in cages with unfamiliar pups, then subjected to several stress situations and observed for maternal behavior. In the sieve barrier stress test, kitchen sieves were placed over the pups. The amount of time that the mothers burrowed for their pups was recorded and interpreted as appropriate caretaking behavior. Table 5-1 shows that the lactating mice burrowed for a significantly longer interval in an attempt to retrieve the pups compared to nonlactating mice, even when the pups were not their own. These same mothers were given the shock barrier test. In this test, the mice were exposed to an electric foot grid, which they were required to cross in order to reach their young. The number of times the mothers crossed the grid and the amount of time that they interacted with their young were recorded. Again, the results in Table 5-1 illustrate that the lactating mothers exposed themselves to painful stimuli twice as often as nonlactating mothers in order to interact with their adopted young. These studies suggest that lactation is essential to the establishment of caretaking behavior.

Early maternal-infant bonding also plays an important role in human caretaking behavior. In a series of Guatemalan studies, 60 primiparous women were randomly assigned to three groups.[17] The first group was the early contact group in which mothers were permitted to lay skin-to-skin with their nude infants under a heat panel immediately after delivery. The second group had delayed skin contact; these mothers were permitted the

Table 5-1
The Effect of Lactation on Maternal Behavior in Mice

Test	Group of Mice	
	Lactating	*Nonlactating*
Sieve barrier		
Minutes of burrowing*		
Day 3	4.1	0.5
Day 4	3.8	0.4
Shock barrier		
Number of times crossing toward pups*	8.6	3.5
Minutes spent with pups*	20.1	9.5

*p 0.01
Adapted from Newton et al.[16]

same skin contact with their newborn infants, but only 12 hours postpartum. Mothers in the control group first saw their infants at 12 hours and had no skin contact for the first 24 hours after delivery. This latter practice was a routine procedure for this obstetric hospital. At 36 hours, the mothers in all groups were evaluated for affectionate behavior by an independent observer who did not know the mothers' previous contact experience (Figure 5-1). The results of the study showed that the mothers who had immediate skin contact displayed a significantly greater amount of affectionate behavior. They looked at the face for a long period[18]; they talked, smiled, and fondled their infants more frequently when compared to mothers who had delayed or no skin contact.

Health care teams regularly visited these same Guatemalan women for one year and recorded the frequency of breast-feeding among the three groups at each visit. A greater number of mothers from the early contact group breast-fed their infants during any one visit compared to the group of mothers with no contact for as long as one year after delivery. The implications from both animal and human studies are that the process of maternal-infant bonding is an essential component of appropriate caretaking behavior, and that lactation plays an integral role in establishing and maintaining this relationship.

Lactational Infertility

Lactation in the human involves both physiologic and psychologic components that are integrated via the neuroendocrine axis of the pituitary and mammary glands.[1,19] Sucking by the infant is the neurogenic stimulus that induces the anterior pituitary to secrete prolactin into the blood. Prolactin in turn stimulates the alveolar cells of the mammary gland to produce milk. The sucking response also stimulates the posterior pituitary to release oxytocin, which causes the myoepithelial cells along the glandular ducts to contract, resulting in milk ejection. Emotional factors, such as maternal anxiety, can inhibit the oxytocin reflex, thereby reducing milk availability and further aggravating what already may be a tenuous mother-infant relationship. Therefore, once established, lactation permits a symbiotic relationship between the mother and the child and requires the integration of the infant's behavior with physical, hormonal, and psychologic changes in the mother.

One of the consequences of the altered hormonal status of the mother during breast-feeding is that of lactational infertility. Assuming that the mother does breast-feed her infant, there are several factors that influence postpartum infertility. These include such factors as the time since birth of

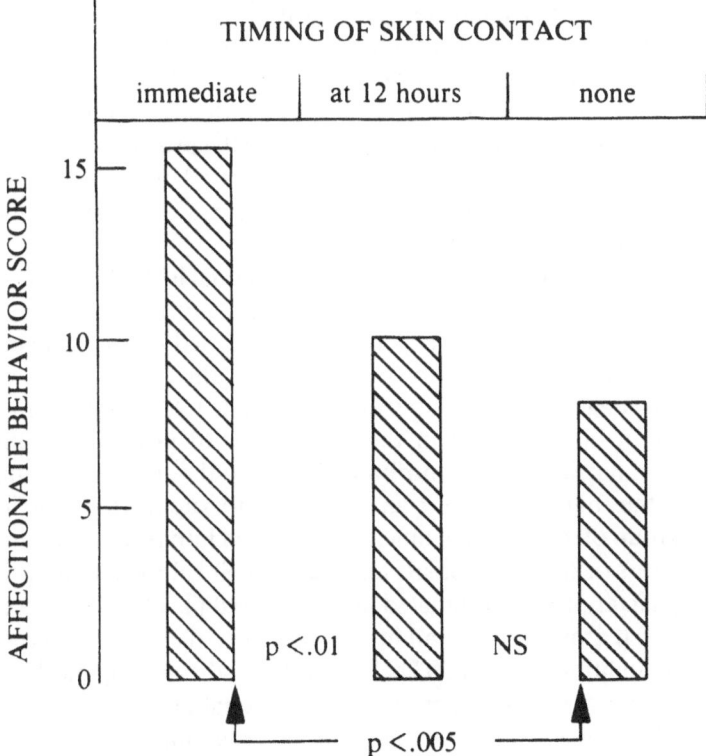

Figure 5-1 Attachment behavior at 36 hours of three groups of mothers who received a different timing of skin contact with their child. Adapted from Sosa et al.[17] Reprinted with permission.

the infant and the intensity, frequency, and duration of nursing. These factors are important because they influence the activity of prolactin, the hormone that plays a significant role in maintaining lactational infertility.[20] Studies indicate that prolactin levels are consistently higher in nursing mothers compared to non-nursing mothers until the 13th postpartum week. Elevated levels of prolactin are also observed after each nursing period, suggesting that frequent feedings promote infertility.

Supplementation with commercial formulas, ie, partial versus complete breast-feeding, also has an effect on the resumption of vaginal bleeding.[20] In one study, mothers at three and one-half months postpartum were divided into two groups: the first group breast-fed their infants entirely, while the second group chose to supplement their infants with other foods, thereby reducing the intensity of nursing. In the supplemented group, vaginal bleeding resumed on an average of 164 days or five and one-half months after delivery, compared to the completely breast-fed group, in which vaginal bleeding resumed on an average of 199 days, or six and one-half months after delivery. The prolactin levels were higher in those women fully breast-feeding than in the supplemented groups. In addition, at the time of the first postpartum menses, higher prolactin levels were associated with proliferative changes on endometrial biopsies, while lower prolactin levels were measured in those women who had secretory changes on their endometrial biopsies. Therefore, it would appear that the protective effects of breast-feeding on conception are mediated by the prolactin levels, which are elevated during lactation. Prolactin in turn regulates gonadal responsiveness to the pituitary gonadotropins. Suppressed ovarian function results in lactational infertility.

One other important factor related to lactational infertility is the nutritional status of the mother. In studies comparing birth intervals, ie, child spacing, between poorly nourished and well-nourished women who breast-fed entirely and used no form of contraception, the delivery of the next child was prolonged in poorly nourished women for 28 months compared to a 22-month birth interval in the well-nourished group of women.[21]

Maternal nutrition also contributes in part to the success or failure of nursing, ie, the ability to produce an adequate milk supply that satisfies the infant. A group of 25 English women were divided into three groups on the basis of success or failure of breast feeding.[22] Their caloric intakes prior to and during lactation were estimated and compared (Table 5-2). Successful mothers ingested at least 500 additional kcal per day over unsuccessful mothers. In addition, at the 500 kcal excess level, the nursing mothers lost weight while those ingesting nearly 1000 additional kcal maintained their weight. In this situation, the well-nourished woman may be infertile for a longer period of time; however, the mechanism that affords this protection is probably related to the greater intensity of nursing and subsequent higher levels of prolactin.

Table 5-2
Effect of Maternal Energy Intakes on the Success or Failure of Breast-Feeding

	Maternal Energy Intakes (kcal/day)	
	Lactating	*Before Lactating*
Successful		
Weight stable	2950	2000
Weight loss	2510	1920
Unsuccessful	1960	1690

Adapted from Whichelow.[22] Reprinted by permission of Cambridge University Press.

Child Development

Many studies have attempted to correlate the mode of infant feeding, either breast or bottle, with the development of the infant through childhood and into adolescence. Needless to say, child development is a complex process that relies not only upon the genetic potential of the individual, but also on the infant's environment. It therefore becomes a challenge to identify parameters of development that can be specifically related in a cause-and-effect manner to the method of feeding during early infancy.

Investigators have evaluated parameters such as oral gratification and activity levels of infants as indicators of the influence of breast-feeding on child development. Applebaum has emphasized that the mechanism of sucking during breast-feeding is very different from that during bottle-feeding.[23] In the former situation, the tongue, when pulling the nipple against the hard palate, draws the areola into the mouth, creating a significant negative pressure. The lips form a C-shaped clamp on the areola-nipple junction, forcing the cheek muslces to contract around the nipple and areola. The gums compress the areola, thereby squeezing milk into the base of the throat. In contrast, during bottle-feeding the rubber nipple strikes the soft palate, frequently causing gagging and interfering with tongue action. Consequently, the tongue moves forward against the gums to control milk flow. The lips are flanged into an O-shape on the nipple, relaxing the cheek muscles. The difference between the sucking mechanisms appears to influence the infant's interest in sucking. Simple techniques such as placing the examiner's finger or a sterile teat in the mouth of an infant and recording the duration of sucking have shown that, after the fourth day, breast-fed infants display more interest by sucking longer and with greater vigor compared to bottle-fed infants.[24,25]

The activity level of infants on arousal from sleep has been another useful parameter to demonstrate the relationship between child development and the mode of infant feeding. Arousal patterns that describe activities such as sucking, eye movements, crying, and limb or whole body movements are associated with developmental maturation. When comparing breast- and bottle-fed infants, observers noted that breast-fed infants displayed a greater level of arousal.[26] They were more alert and displayed a greater amount of body activity compared to bottle-fed infants.

Investigators have also attempted to correlate long-term sucking habits with respect to the duration of breast-feeding. More than 3000 Swedish children were evaluated for long-term sucking habits.[27] Forty percent of these children continued to finger- or dummy-suck at 4 years of age. Of this group, only 3% were breast-fed longer than six months. Of those children who never developed long-term sucking habits or those who terminated these habits before 4 years of age, only 4% were breast-fed longer than six months. From these findings, breast-feeding does not appear to influence long-term sucking habits; however, such behavior is influenced by multiple environmental factors.

Developmental milestones were considered to be factors that might be influenced in part by the method of feeding during infancy. One study conducted in the late 1920s classified nearly 400 children on the basis of feeding method and the duration such methods were utilized.[28] The Stanford-Binet Intelligence Test and the Pinter Patterson Performance Test were administered to these children, while the details of developmental milestones were collected from early records kept by parents and physicians. The results from this study indicated that there was no difference in IQ, performance quotient, or age of dentition when comparing the breast-and bottle-fed groups of children (Table 5-3). However, children who were bottle-fed walked and talked later than those who were breast-fed, regardless of the duration of breast-feeding.

In another study, a speech survey was carried out in 134 5- to 6-year-old children in New Zealand in an attempt to examine the influence of early feeding methods on speech development.[29] The findings from this study indicated that breast-feeding was associated with advanced speech characteristics; clarity of speech, tonal quality, and reading ability were notably improved in breast-fed children when compared to bottle-fed children. This was felt to be the result of accelerated development of the neuromuscular system involved in speech, which was evoked by suckling from the breast.

Behavior patterns of 5- to 6-year-old children were also analyzed in relation to early feeding experiences.[30] Twenty-four children in kindergarten were observed by their teachers and by individuals trained in behavioral testing. The behavior patterns observed in these children were given ratings on a social adjustment scale. The details of feeding habits were obtained from early records kept by the parents and physicians. The

Table 5-3
Developmental Milestones of Breast- and Bottle-Fed Children

Milestones	Mode of Feeding	
	Bottle	*Breast*
Quotient scores		
Intelligence	102	102
Performance	122	125
Developmental milestones (months)		
Dentition	7.5	7.4
Walking	14.7	12.9
Talking	15.2	13.7

Adapted from Hoefer and Hardy: *JAMA* 92:615−619, copyright 1929, American Medical Association.

feeding patterns of these children included four groups: those who were never breast-fed, those in whom nursing was terminated within the first few months of life, those who were supplemented with commercial formulas, and those who were successfully breast-fed for four to six months. The conclusions drawn from these observations showed that the successful and short-term breast-fed groups had the most desirable behavior. These children were most popular with other children, showed the most friendliness toward adults, and took the most responsibility. The group never breast-fed tended to disturb other children at work or play, while both the supplemented and never–breast-fed groups were more inclined to show off and act silly. Needless to say, this was a small group of children who were rated by a complex scoring system. The behaviors seen in these children were no doubt composites of many factors, both individually and socially determined. Again, for these same reasons it is difficult to separate cause and effect with respect to breast-feeding and behavior.

Even more difficult to interpret are those studies that attempt to correlate early feeding experiences with late adolescence and early adult behavior. For example, the security levels of college students were measured by standardized psychologic tests and the results were correlated with the type of early feeding experiences.[31] The results of these tests showed that the highest security levels were obtained by students who were never breast-fed, those who were nursed for less than three months, and those who were breast-fed longer than 12 months.

Another group of college students was given the IPAT Anxiety Scale Performance Test and the Eysenck Personality Inventory for neurotic and extrovert behavior in an attempt to show a relationship between these personality traits and early feeding experiences.[32] Results from these tests showed that the students who were breast-fed longer than six months had the least evidence of anxiety; there was no correlation between breast-feeding and neurotic or extrovert behavior.

While the studies herein suggest some associations between the method of early infant feeding and child development, most investigators would agree that feeding methods do not have reliable and consistent effects on behavioral development.[33] This conclusion prevails due to the collection of unreliable data in the form of retrospective reports and the absence of control groups in terms of feeding schedules, the nutritional satisfaction of each group of infants, the duration of the sucking experience, the matching of groups on the socioeconomic level, or the differences in maternal care and social interaction between mother and infant. Many factors may not be the same in any two groups and any combination of these factors could contribute to differences in child development.

Conclusion

In summary, the following points have been made:

1. Lactation is the natural means by which maternal-infant bonding and caretaking behavior are established. Animal mothers that are separated from their young during the early postpartum period fail to establish appropriate caretaking of their newborn offspring when reintroduced. In contrast, lactating animals perform their mothering duties with more vigor and intensity compared to nonlactating animals. Similarly, in humans, mothers having early contact with their newborn infants displayed a greater amount of affectionate behavior when interacting with their infants. A greater number of early-contact mothers were also breast-feeding at any point in time. These findings have implications regarding problems of maternal deprivation and child abuse.

2. Lactational infertility is an immediate consequence of parturition and its maintenance is related in part to the frequency, intensity, and duration of breast-feeding. The mechanism of infertility is attributed to elevated prolactin levels measured during the postpartum period. Prolactin levels remain elevated with frequent and prolonged nursing, particularly when this method of feeding provides the sole source of nutrition for the infant. The implications of these observations are related to the use of breast-feeding as a natural method for birth control in the general population.

3. The effects of lactation on child development show inconsistent results due to poor study designs and unreliable data collection. Some studies suggest that breast-fed infants are advanced in areas such as early maturation and developmental milestones when compared to bottle-fed infants, while personality traits are variable. In all instances, child development is a multifactorial experience that depends not only on the biologic constitution of the individual but also on the environmental factors that

modify the basic character. The effects of lactation on child development can be interpreted only after careful control of the environmental factors.

REFERENCES

1. Jelliffe DB, Jelliffe EFP: "Breast is best": modern meanings. *N Engl J Med* 297:912–915, 1977.
2. Jenness R: The composition of milk, in Larson BL, Smith VR (eds): *Lactation,* vol 3. New York, Academic Press, 1974, pp 3–107.
3. Guall GE, Rassin DK, Räihä NCR, et al: Milk protein quantity and quality in low birth weight infants. *J Pediatr* 90:348–355, 1977.
4. Rassin DK, Gaull GE, Räihä NCR, et al: Milk protein quantity and quality in low birth weight infants. *J Pediatr* 90:356–360, 1977.
5. Hambraeus L: Proprietary milk versus human milk in infant feeding. *Pediatr Clin North Am* 24:17–36, 1977.
6. Filer LJ Jr, Mattson FH, Fomon SJ: Triglyceride configuration and fat absorption by the human infant. *J Nutr* 99:293–298, 1969.
7. Gyorgy P: Biochemical aspects. *Am J Clin Nutr* 24:970–975, 1971.
8. Saarinen UM, Siimes MA, Dallman PR: Iron absorption in infants: high bioavailability of breast milk iron as indicated by the extrinsic tag method of iron absorption and by the concentration of serum ferritin. *J Pediatr* 91:36–39, 1977.
9. Eckhert CD, Sloan MV, Duncan JR, et al: Zinc binding: a difference between human and bovine milk. *Science* 195:789–790, 1977.
10. Robinson M: Infant morbidity and mortality. *Lancet* 1:788–794, 1951.
11. Cunningham AS: Morbidity and mortality in breast-fed and artificially fed infants. *J Pediatr* 90:726–729, 1977.
12. Goldman AS, Smith CW: Host resistance factors in human milk. *J Pediatr* 82:1082–1090, 1973.
13. Klaus MH, Kennell JH: Human maternal and paternal behavior, in Klaus MH, Kennell JH (eds): *Maternal Infant Bonding.* St. Louis, CV Mosby Co, 1976, pp 38–98.
14. Trause MA, Klaus MH, Kennell JH: Maternal behavior in mammals, in Klaus MH, Kennell JH (eds): *Maternal Infant Bonding.* St. Louis, CV Mosby Co, 1976, pp 16–37.
15. Moore AU: Effects of modified maternal care in the sheep and goat, in Newton G, Levine S (eds): *Early Experience and Behavior.* Springfield, Ill, Charles C Thomas, 1968, pp 481–529.
16. Newton N, Peeler D, Rawlins C: Effect of lactation on maternal behavior in mice with comparative data on humans. *J Reprod Med* 1:257–262, 1968.
17. Sosa R, Kennell JH, Klaus MH, et al: The effect of early mother-infant contact on breast feeding, infection and growth, in Elliott K, Fitzsimons DW (eds): *Breast Feeding and the Mother.* Elsevier, Netherlands, Mouton Publishers, 1976, pp 179–193.
18. Klaus MH, Jerauld R, Kreger NC, et al: Maternal attachment: importance of the first post partum days. *N Engl J Med* 286:460–463, 1972.
19. Schams D: Hormonal control of lactation, in Eliott K, Fitzsimons DW (eds): *Breast Feeding and the Mother.* Elsevier, Netherlands, Mouton Publishing, 1976, pp 27–43.
20. Tyson JE, Freedman RS, Perez A, et al: Significance of the secretion of

human prolactin and gonadotropin for puerperal lactational infertility, in Elliott K, Fitzsimons DW (eds): *Breast Feeding and the Mother*. Elsevier, Netherlands, Mouton Publishing, 1976, pp 49–71.

21. Short RV: Lactation – the control of reproduction, in Elliott K, Fitzsimons DW (eds): *Breast Feeding and the Mother*. Elsevier, Netherlands, Mouton Publishing, 1976, pp 73–86.

22. Whichelow MJ: Success and failure of breast feeding in relation to energy intake. *Proc Nutr Soc* 35:62A–63A, 1976.

23. Applebaum RM: The modern management of successful breast feeding. *Pediatr Clin North Am* 17:203–224 1970.

24. Davis HV, Sears RR, Miller HC, et al: Effects of cup, bottle and breast feeding on oral activities of newborn infants. *Pediatrics* 2:549–558, 1948.

25. Bernal J, Richards MPM: The effects of bottle and breast feeding on infant development. *J Psychosom Res* 14:247–252, 1970.

26. Bell RQ: Level of arousal in breast-fed an bottle-fed human newborns. *Psychosom Med* 28:177–180, 1966.

27. Larsson E: Dummy- and finger-sucking habits in 4-year-olds. *Sven Tandläk Tidsk* 68:219–224, 1975.

28. Hoefer C, Hardy MC: Later development of breast fed and artificially fed infants. *JAMA* 92:615–619, 1929.

29. Broad FE: The effects of infant feeding on speech quality. *NZ Med J* 76:28–31, 1972.

30. Newton NR: The relationship between infant feeding experience and later behavior. *J Pediatr* 38:28–40, 1951.

31. Maslow AH, Szilagyi-Kessler I: Security and breast feeding. *J Abnormal Psychol* 41:83–85, 1946.

32. Hughes RN, Bushnell JA: Further relationships between the IPAT Anxiety Scale Performance and infantile feeding experiences. *J Clin Psychol* 33:698–700, 1977.

33. Caldwell BM: The effects of infant care, in Hoffman ML, Hoffman LW (eds): *Review of Child Development Research,* vol 1. New York, Sage Publications Inc, 1964.

6 Infant Formula — Clinical Evaluation, Its Uses, and Current Feeding Practices in the United States and Developing Countries

Angel Cordano, MD, MPH

In industrialized countries infants are being fed in a variety of ways with very similar results in their growth, development, and health. For most full-term newborns, breast-feeding is considered the ideal method when the mother wants to nurse and is capable of providing adequate amounts of milk for the infant's normal growth. Unfortunately, many women, particularly those from developing countries, may not be adequately nourished and may not provide enough breast milk to meet the infant's total nutrient needs by the third or fourth month.

Supplemental iron, vitamin D, and fluoride are recommended in infants who are breast-fed as their total diet up to 5 or 6 months of life. Fomon[1] has estimated that the infant needs to absorb 200 mg of iron during the first year of life in order to assure an adequate iron nutritional status. This requires an average daily absorption of 0.55 mg. McMillian et al[2] reported that the iron in human milk is uniquely absorbed, assuring good iron status for infants breast-fed for their first six months. Human milk has a concentration of 0.5 mg iron per liter that is about 50% bioavailable, resulting in absorption of only 0.25 mg/day, which would not be sufficient. A proclaimed argument against iron supplementation of breast-fed infants is the increased risk of infection that may result when lactoferrin and transferrin are saturated with iron with reduced bacteriostatic action. These in vitro data have no confirmation of clinical relevance. According to the Committee on Nutrition of the American Academy of Pediatrics,[4] "The benefits of supplementations seem to outweigh the possibility of iron excess during a period of development characterized by marginal stores." Furthermore, unpublished data show that the amount of iron in iron-fortified formulas is not sufficient to saturate the lactoferrin and transferrin.[5] The American Academy of Pediatrics recommends iron supplementation of breast- and formula-fed infants not later than 4 months of age in full-term infants and after 2 months of age in prematures.

Human milk has been thought to be low in vitamin D. However, the report from Lakdawala and Widdowson[6] indicated that human milk contains considerable amounts of an aqueous form of vitamin D-sulfate not measured by previous assay methods. Whether this water-soluble form of vitamin D has the same biologic activity has not yet been determined. There is still much controversy on vitamin D supplementation. The fluoride content of human milk is low even in milk from mothers in fluoridated-water areas. A supplement of 0.25 mg F/day is recommended for breast-fed infants. Supplementation in formula-fed infants depends on the fluoride content of the prepared formula.

In 1976 the Committee on Nutrition of the American Academy of Pediatrics[7] endorsed breast-feeding, but it also stated, "When breast-feeding is unsuccessful, inappropriate, or stopped early, infant formulas provide the best alternative for meeting nutritional needs during the first year."

In the United States about 50% of infants are initially breast-fed, and by six months less than 25% of the infants are either partially or totally breast-fed. Exact figures are not well-known, but there does seem to be a trend toward an increase. Since millions of babies in the United States are formula-fed for one reason or another, it is the manufacturer's responsibility to confirm the quality and adequacy of its products by appropriate clinical studies. Human testing is a necessary final step in the evaluation of dietary products. Although biochemical and animal studies are good predictors of, for example, protein quality, they do not always presage the results of human studies. The adequacy of a diet can only be determined by prolonged feeding of that diet in the target population. As with animal studies, the repletion of the malnourished individual provides a strict biologic assay. Therefore, metabolic balance studies, plasma amino acid analysis, and long-term growth and consumption studies are performed with new formulations before marketing.

Clinical Studies

Metabolic balance studies are conducted in normal newborn infants during the first month of life, with two periods of urine and feces collection of at least three days each. Nitrogen, fat, and selected mineral balances (ie, Zn, P, or Ca) are done. Determinations of nitrogen and fat in feces compared with intake permits calculation of the absorption of these nutrients. Measuring nitrogen in urine allows determination of nitrogen retention, which indicates the quality of the protein of the study product. Occasionally, if newborns are not available, these metabolic balances are conducted in older infants.

When a new protein source or combination of protein sources are utilized, nitrogen balances at levels close to a growing human's minimal requirement (ie, 6.4% calories as protein) are performed. In this type of study four infants are usually studied, each serving as his own control. The control diet is based on casein because of its high quality as a reference protein. Vegetable oil and sugar are added to the study product as a source of calories to achieve a level of 6.4% calories from protein. Nitrogen balance studies at this protein level increase the chance of identifying differences of protein quality between casein and the study product. Fasting, three- and four-hour postprandial plasma aminograms, total protein, and albumin are determined after nine days on each diet.

112-day growth study Fifteen normal newborns of the same sex whose mothers elect not to breast-feed are started on the new formula product during the first week of life. Formula intake and tolerance are determined, as well as gain in weight and growth. Solid foods are not encouraged and their intake is recorded. Height and weight measurements are taken at periodic intervals (ie, 8, 14, 28, 42, 56, 84, and 112 days of age).[8]

Acceptance and tolerance About 100 normal newborn infants whose mothers cannot or elect not to breast-feed are enrolled in these studies. Formula is started the first week of life and continued for three to six months. Volume of formula intake, gastrointestinal tolerance, stool characteristics, and other observations are recorded. A corresponding control group of 100 infants is observed receiving a marketed product. Monthly measurements of height and weight are obtained. Often these studies also include spaced determinations of selected biochemical and hematologic parameters.

Marketing of the new product requires it to perform comparably to or better than currently available products. Standardized growth curves of breast-fed infants are also utilized for comparison of product performance.

Development of Special Infant Formulas

Several developments around the turn of the century made bottle-feeding based on cow's milk more feasible and safer. These included: 1) sanitary handling of milk; 2) heat treatment that produced a sterile evaporated milk, which reduced curd tension; and 3) the addition of carbohydrate to diluted milk, which resulted in better tolerance by the infants. These modified cow's milk formulas preceded the development of current infant formulas that simulate human milk. Reducing the protein and electrolytes, replacing butter fat with vegetable oils, and adding vitamins and minerals essential for the infant, resulted in commercial infant formulas more similar in composition to human milk. An iron-fortified, commercially prepared formula is considered a nutritionally complete food for infants. Figure 6-1 shows how alternate sources of protein, carbohydrate, and fat are used to prepare formulas for the special needs of infants. In 1929 the first soy-based formula (called Sobee) was introduced for feeding allergic infants. Since then, continued improvements in methods of soy protein isolation have permitted development of more elegant soy-based infant formulas. Today, lactose-free soy isolate formulas are also commonly used for infants who temporarily cannot tolerate lactose due to diarrhea or other gastrointestinal illnesses.

Other milk-substitute formulas are available for patients who are not only allergic to milk but cannot assimilate ingredients of soy formulas. An example is Nutramigen, which is a product resulting from an enzymatically digested casein also treated with charcoal to reduce allergenicity. It provides free amino acids and small peptides and is lactose-free. It has been marketed since 1942. A formula based on beef heart (MBF) is another available milk-substitute product for use by infants intolerant to milk. Any of these lactose-free products are also useful in the management of infants suffering from galactosemia.

In recent years elemental diets such as Vivonex and Pregestimil have been utilized in infants with severe gastrointestinal problems, either as a major or total source of nutrition for prolonged periods, or as a transitional feeding when infants are being weaned from total parenteral nutrition. For infants with inborn errors of amino acid metabolism, special diets have been developed. An example is Lofenalac, a product for infants who suffer from phenylketonuria.

Uses of Commercially Prepared Formulas and Cow's Milk

In 1975, Fomon[10] reported breast-feeding was relatively uncommon in the United States with most infants fed commerically prepared formula during the first few months of life. The incidence of breast-feeding declined

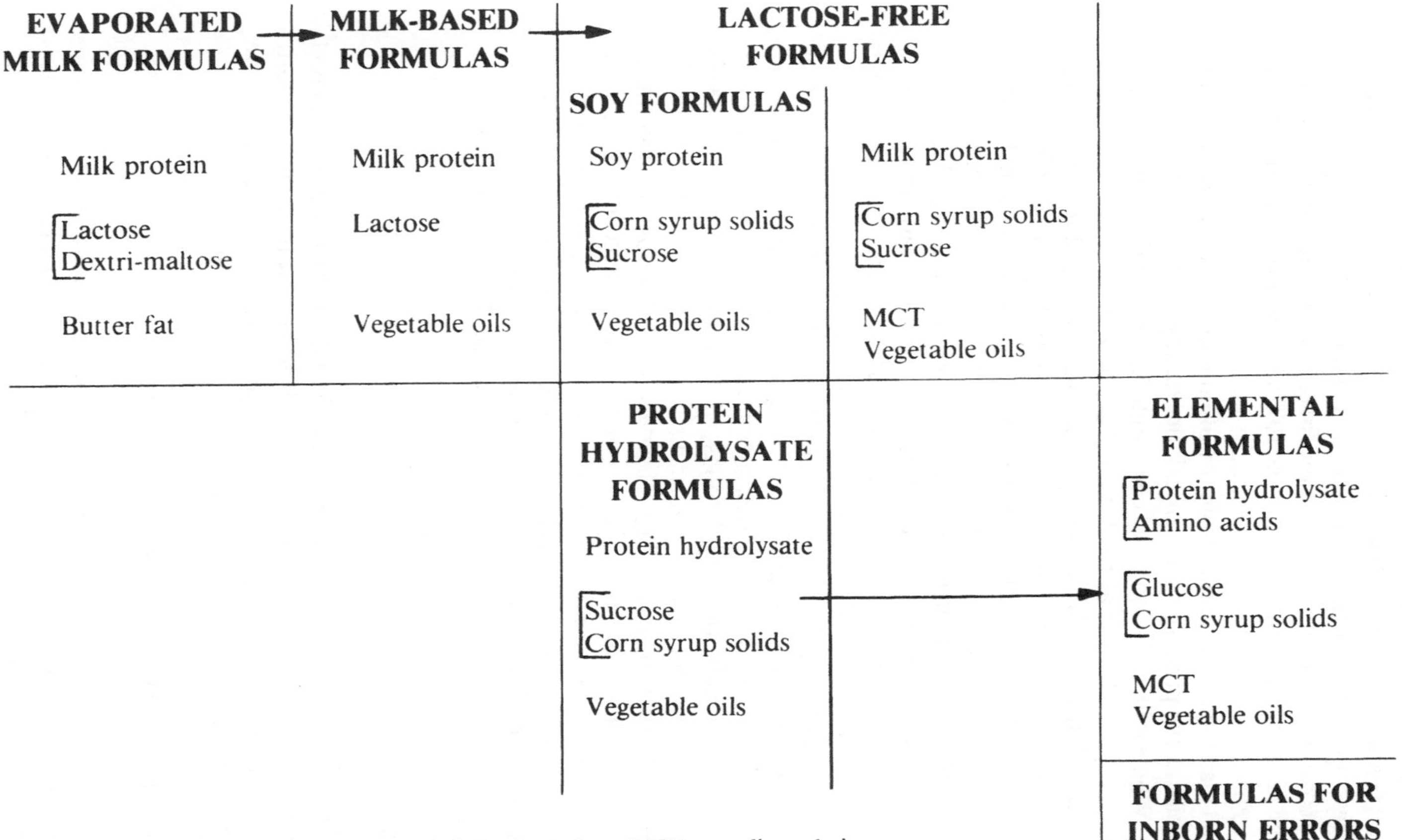

Figure 6-1 Development of special infant formulas. MCT: medium-chain triglycerides. Reprinted from Sarett[9], with permission.

from 20% during the first month to 5% in the fifth month. Milk-based and milk-free commercially prepared formulas accounted for about 75% of the infant feedings. As use of these formulas decreased with increasing age, use of fresh cow's milk increased (Table 6-1). Fomon also found solid foods were commonly introduced during the first month of life. Owen, a member of the panel of nutrition experts at the 1977 telecast program "Infant Nutrition Foundation for Lasting Health,"[11] also discussed the possible nutritional inadequacies resulting from use of unmodified whole, skim, or low-fat milk as the primary source of calories during the first year.

Whole milk   Unmodified cow's milk has several deficiencies making it inappropriate for use as a substantial portion of the infant's nutrient intake. It is high in protein and sodium, contains a poorly absorbed fat, and is inadequate in vitamins C and E as well as iron. It also can cause intolerance in allergic infants.[13,14] Unless heat-treated, it may result in occult blood loss in many infants during the first few months of life.[15] Evaporated cow's milk when properly diluted or whole cow's milk may be acceptable as a portion of the infant's diet during the last part of the first year. However, most pediatric nutritionists recommend continued use of iron-fortified formula until 1 year of age for those infants not breast-fed.

Skim milk   This has all the problems associated with use of whole cow's milk and more. Its calorie supply is insufficient and does not provide essential fatty acids. Fomon and Ziegler in 1977 reported that, when infants received skim milk plus solid foods ad libitum, they consumed large volumes of food but suffered caloric inadequacy with an intake of approximately 80 kcal/kg/day. They observed that skin-fold measurements decreased with use of such a diet, suggesting that a depletion of fat stores was occurring.[16] Bad eating habits may develop due to prolonged ingestion of large volumes of low-calorie feedings. Likewise, the use of low-fat or 2% milk may contribute to unsound eating habits because of the need to consume relatively large volumes to compensate for its caloric density.[12]

Solid Foods

Solid foods should not be started before the baby has achieved good neuromuscular control of his head and neck and is able to sit with support. This occurs between 4 and 6 months of age. At that age most infants are capable of accepting or rejecting the offered solid food.[12]

Low-Birth-Weight Nutritional Requirements

The nutritional requirements for the rapidly growing, small premature infant are higher for many nutrients than for the full-term infant. This is particularly true for calories, protein, calcium, and sodium.

57

Table 6-1
Estimated Percentages of Infants Receiving Various Types of Milks and Formulas

Feeding	Age (mo)							
	0 to 1	1 to 2	2 to 3	3 to 4	4 to 5	5 to 6	6 to 9	9 to 12
Breast-fed	20	15	12	10	8	5	2	1
Milk-based formulas*	64	65	59	49	41	28	3	1
Milk-free formulas*	10	10	10	10	8	6	2	1
Evaporated milk formulas	4	4	3	0	0	0	0	0
Evaporated milk and water	0	0	2	2	2	2	1	1
Fresh cow's milk	2	6	14	29	41	58	92	96

*Commercially prepared.
Adapted from Fomon.[10] Copyright American Academy of Pediatrics 1975.

Table 6-2
Estimated Caloric Intake (kcal/day) From Milk Formulas by Male Infants

Age (mo)	50th Percentile	Calories (% of Total)
0 to 1	400	93
1 to 2	565	85
2 to 3	625	70
3 to 4	640	67
4 to 5	675	64
5 to 6	740	60
6 to 9	820	45
9 to 12	925	34

Adapted from Fomon[10]. Copyright American Academy of Pediatrics 1975.

Premature infants are fed quite differently by different people. Some use fresh or pooled human milk; others recommend prepared infant formulas or special formulas prepared for the low—birth-weight infants. These tailored premature formulas have a higher protein and calorie content, medium-chain triglycerides as a partial source of fat, and a mixture of lactose and corn syrup solids with relatively low osmolalities.

Fomon and Ziegler[17] stated in 1977 that under some circumstances human milk may be nutritionally inadequate and small premature infants could be at risk of developing deficiencies of specific nutrients. Their calculations were restricted to the period during which the infant gains 1160 to 1830 g. Table 6-3 summarizes their calculations, which led to the conclusion that per unit of energy, concentrations of protein, calcium and sodium in human milk are inadequate for growing premature infants. Although not included in the table, our calculations suggest that the content of several other minerals in human milk is also inadequate for growing premature infants. Thus, if human milk is to be used as a food for such infants, it seems

Table 6-3
Protein, Calcium, and Sodium Requirements for
Growing Premature Infants (1160 to 1830 g)

	Protein (g/100 kcal)	Calcium (mg/100 kcal)	Sodium (mEq/100 kcal)
Requirement*	2.54	132	2.3
Composition of banked human milk	1.50	43	0.8

*Assumed body weight is 1200 g; weight gain, 20 g/day; energy intake 120 kcal/kg/day.
Adapted from Fomon and Ziegler: *Am J Dis Child* 131:463, 1977. Copyright 1977, American Medical Association.

reasonable to consider supplementation with protein and minerals. Such consideration should not be undertaken lightly because of the theoretically based possibility that amino acid imbalance or toxicity, acidosis, or other adverse consequences may result.[17]

Fomon and Ziegler clearly state that feeding premature infants with human milk is not to be abandoned, and in fact state that for the ill premature infant or the one unable to ingest enough calories to permit growth, feedings that provide much more protein and minerals than human milk may be desirable.

Breast-Feeding–Infant-Formula Controversy in the Developing World

One of the most bitter controversies in the past few years has been in relation to the declining incidence of breast-feeding and the marketing of formulas in developing countries. Many critics of formula manufacturers reason that the decline of breast-feeding and high rates of infant mortality are due to the availability of prepared infant formula products, and the fact that they are used in many impoverished societies where the lack of clean water supply and adequate sanitation are clearly evident. In 1973, Raphael, Director of the Human Lactation Center, stated[18] "A growing trend away from breast-feeding infants and toward the use of artificial milk is resulting in increased malnutrition and death." In April 1978 she made the following comment on this earlier declaration: "This was an unscientific and inaccurate statement from an individual assuming an advocate's role based on the statement of others and her own limited impressions." She also said that the "Center now questions the assumption of any group which would suggest the elimination of any commercial infant foods on the yet unverifiable theory that they harm babies." She indicated that the effects of poverty, lack of food and safe drinking water, the absence of sanitation and health care, and political indifference to mothers in poverty are the principal determinants of disease and death of infants in the developing world.[19]

Infant morbidity and mortality are correlated with poverty, as child health is associated with affluence. These findings have been correlated by many investigators for over the past 50 years. Infant mortality in developing societies had decreased over the last three decades until 1973, when food prices began to escalate. Only a few countries have data available after 1973, eg, Chile, where the decline continues from 65.2 per 1000 births in 1973 to 54 per 1000 births in 1976 (Monckeberg, personal communication, 1978).

Breast milk is the preferred food for the infant during the early months of life, but breast-feeding exclusively for many undernourished mothers in the less developed countries may provide inadequate nutrition for the growing infant beyond the baby's third or fourth month. Most infants require supplementation with formula or solids thereafter.

60

In summary we can say that: 1) Breast-feeding is preferred as the first choice for most infants when available and appropriate. 2) Extended breast-feeding or feeding with an iron-fortified infant formula is recommended for the first year. 3) Delayed introduction of solid foods until the baby is 4 to 6 months old is recommended. In developing countries, a formula or supplement of good quality should be started around the third or fourth month in infants of malnourished mothers. 4) Infant formula is the best available alternative for most babies who are not breast-fed during the first year. 5) Adequate clinical studies should be conducted with new formulations to ensure they are meeting the infant's growth requirements.

REFERENCES

1. Fomon SJ: *Infant Nutrition*, ed 2. Philadelphia, WB Saunders Co, 1974.
2. McMillian J, Oski FA, Lourie G, et al: Iron Absorption from human milk, simulated human milk and proprietary formulas. *Pediatrics* 60:876, 1977.
3. Saarinen UM, Siimes MA, Dallman PR: Iron absoprtion in infants: high bioavailability of breast milk iron as indicated by the extrinsic tag method of iron absorption and by the concentration of serum ferritin. *J Pediatr* 91:36, 1977.
4. Committee on Nutrition: Relationship between iron status and incidence of infection in infancy. *Pediatrics* 62:247, 1978.
5. Silverio J: Letter to the Editor. Comments on Nutritional Committee statements. *Pediatrics* 61:673, 1978.
6. Lakdawala DR, Widdowson EM: Vitamin D in human milk. *Lancet* 1:167, 1977.
7. American Academy of Pediatrics, Committee on Nutrition: Commentary on breast-feeding and infant formulas, including proposed standards for formulas. *Pediatrics* 57:278, 1976.
8. Fomon SJ, Thomas LN, Filer LJ Jr, et al: Food consumption and growth of normal infants fed milk-based formulas. *Acta Peadiatr Scand [Suppl]* 223:1971.
9. Sarett HP: Special sources of nutrients in dietary management of gastrointestinal disease. *Compr Ther* 4(10):18–23, 1978.
10. Fomon SJ: What are infants fed in the United States? *Pediatrics* 56:350, 1975.
11. Filer J (chairman): *Infant Nutrition Foundation for Lasting Health.* Telecast by Health Learning Systems Inc, 1977.
12. Barness LA: *Dialogues in Infant Nutrition* 1(2): 1977.
13. Owen G. Lippman G: Nutritional status of infants and young children: USA. *Pediatr Clin North Am* 24(1):211, 1977.
14. Woodruff CW: The science of infant nutrition and the art of infant feeding. *JAMA* 240:657, 1978.
15. Wilson JF, Lahey ME, Heiner DC: Studies on iron metabolism. V. Further observations on cow's milk-induced gastrointestinal feeding in infants with iron deficiency anemia. *J Pediatr* 84:335–344, 1974.
16. Fomon SJ, Ziegler EE: *Skim Milk in Infant Feeding.* Rockville, Md, US Departments of Health, Education and Welfare, Public Health Service, Health Services Administration, and Bureau of Community Health Services, 1977.
17. Fomon SJ, Ziegler EE: Human milk and the small premature infant. *Am J Dis Child* 131:463, 1977.

18. Raphael DR: The role of breast-feeding in a bottle-oriented world, in Raphael DR (ed): *Ecology of Food and Nutrition,* vol 2. Westport, Conn, The Human Lactation Center, Ltd, 1973.

19. Raphael DR: *The Lactation Review* 111(1): 1978.

7 Breast- Versus Bottle-Feeding: Psychological Outcome

Esther Wender, MD

Two recent articles report an association, presumably causal, between bottle-feeding and, in the first paper,[1] an increase in learning disorders, and, in the second paper,[2] a generally lower academic performance. In both studies the comparison was with a group of breast-fed infants. One implication of these studies is that nutritional factors, presumably higher concentration of protein in cow's milk formula, result in decreased academic performance. The findings of these studies add to the mounting enthusiasm for a return to breast-feeding as the primary source of nutrition for all infants. Evidence for the potential advantage of breast-feeding is most easily and reliably obtained from investigations that directly analyze differences in the nutrient and biological activity of breast milk compared to cow's milk formula. However, once those differences are verified, they must be shown to relate to different outcomes in the health or development of children. If such a relationship cannot be established, the biological analysis would be unimportant. This need to correlate basic findings with clinical outcome has led to several studies in recent years comparing the later health and/or psychological performance of infants that are exclusively fed breast milk and those exclusively fed formula derived from cow's milk.

In the first part of this chapter I shall review the two recent studies referred to above. Though other psychological outcome studies appear in the literature, all are fraught with such obvious methodological problems that they are not, in my opinion, worthy of close consideration. In the second part of this chapter I shall discuss some of the basic methodological problems encountered in this type of outcome study — that is, the difficulty in establishing comparable groups of breast-fed and formula-fed infants because the type of feeding involves personal choice, a factor which introduces significant bias into the selection of patient samples. Several studies provide evidence of factors that enter into choice of feeding, and these will be reviewed. Finally, I shall conclude with my opinion regarding the relationship between type-of-feeding choices and psychological outcome in infants which will, hopefully, be of some help to the nutritional clinician.

The first study was conducted by Menkes et al and reported in 1977. The study population consisted of 29 children seen in the private practice of a pediatric neurologist and referred because of a learning disorder. The infant feeding histories of this group were compared to a control group of the same age and sex, belonging to the same private practice but referred for other neurological problems. In this control group of 53 children, 27 had a seizure disorder, 7 complained of chronic headache, and 19 had a variety of other neurological problems. Some of the children in the control group also had learning problems, but this was not the primary complaint. Eliminated from the study were all pre-term infants and all who had illnesses that might affect feeding choice. The study population was homogeneous, consisting entirely of white children from families belonging to social classes 1 and 2 (Drillien). This author defined "breast-fed" as "nursed for four weeks or longer." According to the feeding histories obtained on these two populations, 13.8% of the group referred for learning disorders had been breast fed compared to 47.2% of the control group, a difference which was statistically significant.

It is Menkes' et al[2] hypothesis that differences in complex intellectual processes may be produced by the high levels of tyrosine frequently noted in the newborn period in all infants, but with much greater prevalence in infants fed formulas high in protein concentration. This tyrosinemia is apparently due to a transient defect of tyrosine metabolism, a defect which correlates with gestational age; that is, the younger the gestational age, the more severe and prolonged the defect in tyrosine metabolism. The following is a comparison of protein concentration in human breast milk compared to cow's milk and cow's-milk-based formulas: in grams per liter, breast milk contains 9 g, cow's milk 35 g and the most popular formulas contain 15 g of protein. In addition, however, the amino acid composition of breast milk is relatively low in phenylalanine and tyrosine compared to cow's milk.

Investigators[3,4] of this hypothesis provide some evidence that a slight reduction in intellectual and perceptual abilities at school age relates to prolonged, high levels of tyrosine in the neonatal period, and that the prevalence of prolonged high levels of tyrosine in the newborn period is related both to gestational age and to feeding with formulas high in protein concentration.

Because of these speculations, Menkes, in the study described here, also compared the protein content of the formulas fed to the infants in the study population and the controls, but he found no differences between the groups on that parameter.

Following this report by Menkes, there appeared in 1978 a study by Rodgers involving large numbers of children from the National Survey of Health and Development in Great Britain. The survey sample consisted of 5362 live births during one week in 1946. The study was conducted on all children in this sample born to non-manual and agricultural workers, plus a random, 1-in-4 sample of all remaining children. In the original survey there were interviews with the mothers shortly after birth and at 2-year intervals thereafter. These interviews provided information concerning feeding, birthweight, birth rank, social class, and educational attainment of the parents. The survey also provided achievement test data at ages 8, 11, and 15. These tests included a picture vocabulary intelligence test, a test involving reading individual words, a written sentence completion test, a mathematics computation examination, and some kind of assessment of non-verbal ability. Of the total study population, 1133 children were entirely bottle-fed and 1291 were entirely breast-fed. The remainder were fed by combinations of the two. The initial analysis compared test scores in the totally bottle-fed and totally breast-fed groups, and in all instances the breast-fed group had better scores that were statistically significant at the 0.1 level of confidence. However, statistical analyses also demonstrated a relationship between breast-feeding and higher social class, higher educational level in the parent, greater parental interest in education, and children of lower birth rank, all factors which are likely to relate to educational achievement. Therefore, a multiple regression analysis was done to partial out these factors in addition to the type-of-feed variable. When this was done, the differences between the two feeding groups were much smaller, though still statistically significant. The very large number of children studied (2424) meant that, though statistically significant, the differences between the groups were very small.

These two studies — though each has its limitations — provide some evidence that breast feeding may lead to a better psychological outcome, and Menkes suggested a mechanism to explain the differences. One major problem, however, with both studies is whether a population of breast-fed infants can be considered to be comparable — in important ways that may well affect psychologicial outcome — to a group of bottle-fed infants since type of feeding involves something other than random choice. This issue has been competently reviewed recently by Sauls[6] in the October 1979 issue of *Pediatrics*. What I would like to review with you now are some of the variables that have been shown to enter into choice-of-feeding decisions.

In 1960, Brown et al[7] studied 110 primiparas in their third trimester of pregnancy. Of this total group, 55 mothers had chosen breast-feeding and 55 had chosen bottle-feeding. One-half of the group was recruited from a private practice and the other from a clinic that served a generally low socio-economic group. The number that had chosen bottle- or breast-feeding was evenly divided between these two populations. All mothers were at least 16 years old and had IQs between 90 and 110. All had completed at least one year of high school. All were living with their husbands and none had any significant physical or mental disorder. The object of this study was to compare a variety of attitudes that characterized these groups selected on the basis of their choice of type of feeding prior to the lying-in period. The primary measure was a questionnaire that ascertained attitudes toward the chosen feeding method. Table 7-1 lists those attitudes that significantly distinguished between the two groups.

Table 7-1
Infant Feeding By Primiparas*

| | Feeding Group | | |
Results:	*Breast (%)*	*Bottle (%)*	*Significance*
Breast-feeding ties you down	30	57	.01
Bottle more convenient	17	65	.001
Breast-feeding more attractive to husband	30	5	.01
Baby enjoys breast more than bottle	85	35	.001
Breast-feeding makes breasts less attractive	24	42	.05
Breast-feeding may not provide right milk	16	33	.05

*Brown et al, *Psychosom Med* 22:421-9, 1960.

This study provides some evidence for the general conclusion, stated by several authors, that mothers who choose breast-feeding tend to be more *infant*-centered, while mothers who choose bottle-feeding tend to be more *self*-centered. Note, for example, the statement that babies enjoy the breast more than the bottle. Eighty-five percent of the breast-feeding mothers compared to 35% of the bottle-feeding group felt this was true. It is interesting to note that this 35% chose bottle-feeding despite their belief that infants preferred the breast. Note also the big discrepancy between the two groups concerning the statement that the bottle is more convenient. Sixty-five percent of the bottle-feeding group felt this was so, though the only respect in which convenience can be logically associated with bottle-feeding is that with breast-feeding the mother must be present, and, in the eyes of many mothers, breast feeding must take place in privacy.

A second study took place in 1979, and was reported by Switzky et al.[9] This group studied 83 mothers of 6-week-old infants recruited from the private practice of several pediatricians. They selected for study only those mothers who were either exclusively breast-feeding or had exclusively bottle-fed for the 6-week period. Forty-one were in the breast-feeding group and 42 in the bottle-feeding group. The object of this study was to compare attitudes towards parenting in the two groups. The measure used was the Parental Attitude Research Instrument, a questionnaire which yields information in 12 different areas including such categories as: fostering dependence; marital conflict; strictness; rejection or acceptance of homemaking role; suppression or openness of sexuality; and desire to accelerate the child's developmental pace. These authors also administered a feeding questionnaire which asked such questions as whether friends or relatives breast- or bottle-fed, or the husband's attitude toward type of feeding. Those factors that contributed significantly to a differentiation between the groups are listed in Table 7-2.

Table 7-2
Predictors of Breast- /Bottle-Feeding*

Variables contributing significantly to differentation between groups

Higher in breast-fed group:
    Education of mother
    No. of children previously breast-fed
    No. of mother's friends breast-feeding
    Husband's perceived attitude toward breast-feeding
    Mother's overt and covert attitude toward breast-feeding

Higher in bottle-fed group:
    Husband's attitude toward bottle-feeding
    Marital conflict
    Suppression of sexuality
    Acceleration of development

*Switzky et al, *Psychol Rep* 45:3-14, 1979.

Again, this study lends some evidence for the notion that mothers who breast-feed tend to be more infant-oriented. The two groups could be distinguished, for example, on the variable of "acceleration of development", which refers to the mother's desire to have the child grow up more quickly. This group was also able to document an oft said but little documented statement that breast-feeding mothers seem to come from more satisfying marriages. The bottle-fed group experienced a greater amount of marital conflict. The authors speculated that only women who perceive their marriage as well-adjusted choose breast-feeding. This "hunch" is perhaps confirmed by another finding, that breast-feeding mothers perceive their husbands as very supportive of that type of feeding, while bottle-feeding mothers perceive their husband's attitudes as more neutral. It is also of interest, though this difference barely achieved significance, that bottle-feeding mothers scored higher on the suppression-of-sexuality scale. Several less well controlled studies have suggested that bottle-feeding mothers experience greater conflict over the breast as a sexual vs a feeding organ. Evidence for this conflict comes from studies that have shown that bottle-feeding mothers are more likely to disapprove of breast-feeding in public, and have stronger views about the inappropriateness of sexual play in children.

A recent abstract in *Clinical Research* adds further evidence to some of these variables that seem to distinguish between women who choose bottle-/ or breast-feeding in our culture.[10] This 1978 report by Wilson compared a Q-sort done by 20 primiparas who had chosen breast-feeding with 20 who had chosen bottle-feeding. The Q-sort is a technique that encourages the subject to make choices among a large number of words, in this case adjectives that might apply to a person's self-concept, by requiring the subject to rank those words along a bell-shaped curve according to the degree to which they do or do not apply to himself. As an example, consider the 10 adjectives said to characterize the good Boy Scout, ie, brave, truthful, clean, kind, reverent, etc. In a Q-sort the subject might be asked to place the four adjectives most like him in the middle slot, then a cluster of two on either side of the middle, and finally each of the ones least like him at the extreme right or left of the middle. Employing this technique, this group found the following correlations between self-concept and type of feeding choice as shown in Table 7-3.

Table 7-3
Self-Concept in Breast-/Bottle-Feeding Primiparas*

Measures - Q-sort using 48 adjectives
Results†:

Breast-feeders scored higher on:
    Personal aspirations
    Acceptance of others
    Physical self-concept
Breast-feeders:
    Better educated
    More likely employed
    Fewer accidental pregnancies
    Spouses better educated
Bottle-feeders:
    More negative self-concept
    Higher no. of accidental pregnancies

*Wilson et al, *Clin Res* 26:743 A, 1978
†n = 20 in each group.

Note that breast-feeders were not only better educated and had better educated spouses — findings repeatedly confirmed in other studies in our culture — but that breast-feeders also scored higher on positive self-concept, a variable that would seem to strongly influence psychological outcome in the infant and, yet, a variable that has not been considered in the attempt to balance the breast-feeding and bottle-feeding groups compared in psychological outcome studies.

Finally, the work of Klaus and Kennell[12] as it applies to choice of feeding should be briefly reviewed. These investigators have presented provocative evidence that differences in mother-infant interaction when infants are one-month and six-months old, and differences in some test scores at age two can be found when the mother-infant dyads are distinguished only by a period of extended contact between mother and infant in the first two hours after birth. The control group of mother-infant pairs were separated soon after delivery following the usual pattern of care in hospital deliveries, while the study groups were given their infants immediately after delivery for a period of 45 minutes to an hour during which time they were encouraged to breast-feed. Sosa[11] studied the length of time urban Guatemalan mothers continued to breast-feed in a group of mothers who experienced this type of extended contact compared to a control group that did not. Table 7-4 below shows the differences between these groups.

Table 7-4
Duration of Breast-Feeding (in days)*

Number (each group)	Hospital	Control	Experimental	Significance
34	Roosevelt II	109	159	0.1
20	Social Security	104	196	0.05

*Sosa et al *Ciba Found Symp* 451:179-188, 1976

In both studies the experimental group breast-fed for a longer period of time though the only factors that distinguished them from the controls was the extended period of contact immediately after delivery. Interestingly, this difference was more pronounced in the group of uniformly low socioeconomic class. These authors completed a third study that actually demonstrated the reverse of this finding — namely, that the control group breast-fed longer. However, when they analyzed the social class data they found that the experimental and control groups showed significant social class differences, with the control group coming from a higher social class. It is interesting to speculate whether mothers from a higher socioeconomic class are unaffected by the extended contact after birth, or whether mothers in a very low socioeconomic group experience minimal attachment unless they received this type of extended contact. In either case this study provided evidence that type of feeding may be affected by measures designed to increase the strength of the maternal-infant attachment. This finding makes sense in the light of the data already presented regarding the infant-centered tendency in breast-feeding mothers.

What do all of these data have to do with breast- /bottle-feeding outcome studies? In both studies reported here, the authors tried to balance the characteristics of the breast- and bottle-feeding groups on the basis of socioeconomic class, and, in the case of Rodger's study,[5] on the basis of educational level of the mother and parental interest in education. But in neither study were the groups balanced on the basis of infant- vs self-centeredness or degree of perceived marital conflict, both factors which one would expect might also affect psychological outcome.

Despite these obvious limitations I find the results of Menkes's study[2] provocative for two reasons. First, outcome studies based upon comparing groups with documented high or low tyrosine levels in infancy, have demonstrated differences in perceptual function — not in overall IQ — when these children reached school age, and children with learning disability have just that combination of characteristics, ie, normal IQ, but lower scores on perceptual function. Second, learning disability has a strong genetic component and is frequently associated with high levels of tension and anxiety, present even before the learning problem is noticed and, therefore, probably partly temperamental in origin. I wonder if the mothers of learning-disabled children are more likely to share these qualities of tension and anxiety on a genetic basis and, therefore, be poorer risks for successful breast-feeding. In other words, does bottle-feeding produce the learning disability or do the genetic traits shared in LD families lead to a greater likelihood that breast-feeding will not be successful?

What conclusions can be offered to the nutritional clinician? I believe the evidence is much too scanty to allow recommendations in favor of breast-feeding to be made on the basis of a link between breast-feeding and a favorable psychological outcome for the infant. It does seem clear, however, that factors often associated with breast-feeding result in a better academic and psychological outcome in infants fed this way. It seems equally clear that these factors can also be present in bottle-fed babies and can lead to equally favorable chances for later academic and psychological performance. It would agree with the recommendations of Gunther [13] in an interesting paper included in the recent Ciba Foundation Symposium on breast-feeding. She advises that "A mother is helped best by listening and understanding." She goes on to explain that choice-of-feeding decisions in our culture are based on a variety of fairly deep-seated feelings that cannot so easily be affected by simple advice. This conclusion is reinforced by several, rather disheartening, studies that have demonstrated that encouraging breast-feeding in the newborn nursery may increase the number of mothers breast-feeding at the time of hospital discharge, but has almost no effect on the number still breast-feeding six weeks later. How-to-feed decisions are apparently made by most mothers long before the lying-in period.[14] The most hopeful approach, in my opinion, comes from the work on extended contact in the immediate post-delivery period and the effect that procedure may have on several maternal behaviors including the inclination to breast-feed. This approach seems particularly applicable to policies in the urban populations of underdeveloped countries where a recent increase in bottle-feeding seems to have such serious consequences in a culture not ready to handle that change.

Meanwhile, in our culture, we must all continue to tread a careful line between overenthusiasm for breast-feeding, sometimes based upon our own deep-seated values and also based upon the increasing evidence of the intricately balanced nutritional qualities of the milk best designed for human consumption — between that and the danger of producing a mother neurosis stemming from the conflicts experienced by women who want the best for their infants but also experience a genuine dislike for or anxiety concerning the breast-feeding process.

REFERENCES

1. Menkes JH: Early feeding history of children with learning disorders. *Develop Med Child Neurol* 19:169–171, 1977.

2. Menkes JH, Welcher DW, Levi HS, et al: Relationship of elevated blood tyrosine to the ultimate intellectual performance of premature infants. *Pediatrics* 49:218–224, 1972.

3. Mamunes P, Prince PE, Thornton NH, et al: Intellectual deficits after transient tyrosinemia in the term neonate. *Pediatrics* 57:675–680, 1976.

4. Hambraeus L: Proprietary milk versus human breast milk in infant feeding: A critical appraisal from the nutritional point of view. *Symposium on Nutrition in Pediatrics* 24:17–36, 1977.

5. Rodgers B: Feeding in infancy and later ability and attainment: A longitudinal study. *Develop Med Child Neuro* 20:421–426, 1978.

6. Sauls HS: Potential effect of demographic and other variables in studies comparing morbidity of breast-fed and bottle-fed infants. *Pediatrics* 64:523–527, 1979.

7. Brown F, Liberman J, Winston J, et al: Studies in choice of infant feeding in primiparas. *Psychosom Med* 22:421–429, 1960.

8. Newton N: Psychologic differences between breast and bottle feeding. *Am Clin Nut* 24:993–1004, 1971.

9. Switzky LT, Vietze P, Switzsky HN: Attitudinal and demographic predictors of breast-feeding and bottle-feeding behavior by mothers of six week old infants. *Psychol Rep* 45:3–14, 1979.

10. Wilson PL: Self concept of selected breast feeding and bottle feeding primiparas: A pilot exploratory descriptive study. Abstract, *Clin Res* 26:743 A, 1978.

11. Sosa R, Kennell JH, Klaus M, et al: The effect of early mother-infant contact on breast feeding, infection and growth. *Ciba Found Symp.* 451:159, 1976, pp. 179–188.

12. Klaus MH, Jerauld R, Kreger NC, et al: Maternal attachment: importance of the first post-partum days. *N Eng J Med* May 2 1972, pp. 460–463.

13. Gunther M: The new mother's view of herself. *Ciba Found Symp* 451;159, 1976, pp. 145–152.

14. Hollen BK: Attitudes and practices of physicians concerning breast-feeding and its management. *Environ Child Health* December 1976, pp. 288–293.

8 Nutritional Problems of Physically and Mentally Handicapped Children

John M. Carper, MD

About 3% of Americans have mental retardation and developmental problems, of which 3,000,000 are children and adolescents. There are 126,000 babies born each year who will have some degree of mental impairment. Fortunately, for 95% of them the impairment will be minimal to moderate, but those with severe problems will command an inordinate amount of medical care and educational resources.

I would like to review briefly the history of pediatrics and mention some of the diseases that have yielded to medical research, diseases that accounted for much mental retardation a generation or two ago. I would also like to describe the cycle of managing retarded children that has occurred over the past 100 years: from keeping the retarded child at home to placing him in an institution, to the recent swing back to home care.

Pediatrics, among all specialties, has been proud of the advances it has made in the prevention of disease. In fact, pediatrics as a specialty began with the knowledge of infectious diseases and infant feeding. Vaccines were developed against tetanus, diphtheria, and whooping cough, and pediatricians began to immunize infants routinely against these diseases along with smallpox. The epidemiology of tuberculosis, scarlet fever, measles, mumps, rubella, chicken pox, poliomyelitis, and meningitis was understood by the turn of the century and quarantine procedures were instituted, inhibiting their spread to the community. Some of these diseases became treatable with the discovery of antibiotics and chemotherapeutic agents following World War II, and basic research of the 1940s and 1950s led to the discovery and use of effective live viral vaccines for most of the other childhood diseases. Hemolytic disease of the newborn, with its high mortality and almost certain morbidity of deafness, cerebral palsy, and mental retardation in the severely affected survivors, yielded to basic research in blood-group incompatibility and is not only treatable but frequently prevented by RhoGAM injection of susceptible mothers.

By the early 1960s there was a period of euphoria among pediatricians and other professionals concerned with mental retardation and cerebral palsy. The antibiotics and immunization with bacterial and viral vaccines had eliminated broad categories of diseases that in the past were major sources of cerebral palsy and retardation. New understanding of chromosomal disease and amniocentesis promised antenatal diagnosis and therapeutic abortion of the fetus at risk. Dietary control of phenylketonuria was proving effective and other metabolic causes of retardation were hoped to be amenable to similar treatment.

The goal of eliminating cerebral palsy and mental retardation has not yet been realized. Replacing the etiologies described earlier was a byproduct of our increasingly sophisticated knowledge of physiology and the hardware it spawns. Tracheal intubation, open and closed methods of heart stimulation, and improved management of acidosis, fluid, and electrolyte imbalances resulted in the survival of many newborns who formerly would have died. Infant mortality among premature infants and those infants with respiratory distress syndrome has steadily decreased in the past ten years, as knowledge expands and is extended to areas outside university hospitals. The price for this knowledge is a moderate-size group of survivors who have neurologic and cognitive deficits ranging from profound retardation to minimal brain dysfunction and specific learning problems. Impairment of vision, hearing, and motor function is frequently present to a degree. Not all of these children come from newborn nurseries, as resuscitative techniques are also used for the child with severe sepsis or meningitis, who has been severely brain-injured by trauma, or who survives the anoxia caused by an accidental ingestion. Thus medical science "takes away" at the same time it "gives," and it is probable that mental retardation and cerebral palsy will be with us for many generations.

About 100 years ago, as the United States began to change from an agrarian society to an industrial one, the extended family was broken up, and the profoundly retarded, multiply-handicapped child could no longer be managed at home. The state began to build institutions for their custodial care; the Fernald State School in Waltham, Mass. was the first of these in the United States. Located in rural areas, they were largely inaccessible to parents' visits, and services gradually decreased to the minimal level of feeding and care of basic body functions. About 20 years ago, social scientists, psychologists, and pediatricians compared the development of patients with Down's syndrome placed in an institution at birth with those raised at home, and found significant differences of function in favor of those kept at home. This led to the current emphasis on early stimulation of the retarded infant and child in the home and in day-care facilities, and postponement of institutionalization as long as possible.

Massachusetts was a leader in establishing a chapter of its educational code (Chapter 766) that ensured the right of all handicapped children between the ages of 3 and 22 to free, appropriate public education. Public Law 94-142, the Education for All Handicapped Children Act, was passed by the Congress of the United States and went into effect in October 1977. All state and local education agencies are now required to arrange for yearly evaluations of handicapped children and to develop and administer individualized educational programs for these youngsters. Parents are given a role in placement decisions and are empowered with major due-process guarantees in the event they disapprove of placement decisions.

Because it is inevitable that some physicians will soon be called upon for advice by parents or staff concerning feeding and nutrition of these difficult children, I would like to share some of my experiences.

For the past four years, I have been a pediatric consultant to Project EISEC, a day-care facility operated by the Department of Child Psychiatry of Boston University School of Medicine and the Fuller Mental Health Center. EISEC is an acronym for Early Intervention and Stimulation of Exceptional Children. The target population we serve consists of profoundly damaged children 2 to 12 years of age who live in Boston, with a priority to the area served by the Fuller Mental Health Center: Roxbury, South End, North Dorchester, and Back Bay. The highest proportion of welfare patients in the city live in this area. Two-thirds of the population is black and one-fourth is Hispanic. Thirty-five to forty children are enrolled in this program. They live at home and attend classes five days a week from 9:00 AM to 1:30 PM. They are bussed to the school and parents send along a hot lunch. The goals of the project are to provide a day-care setting and educational program for these children, and to provide emotional support for their parents. Various methods are used to improve cognitive skills, prevent contractures, and stimulate all sensory modalities. A profile of the children's handicaps is seen in Table 8-1. Table 8-2 demonstrates the multiple professionals involved in the care of these children.

Table 8-1
Profile of Handicaps in EISEC

Handicap	Percent
Mental retardation	100
Profound	50
Visual impairment	50
Blind	25
Hearing deficit	25
Nonverbal	90
Unable to walk	80
Seizures	75
Spasticity	80
Feeding problems	90

Etiology of the problems of these children includes: prematurity, anoxia, neonatal sepsis, meningitis, child abuse resulting in severe brain injury, congenital rubella and toxoplasmosis, and chromosomal abnormalities.

Table 8-2
Staffing Pattern at EISEC

Teacher
Teacher aides
Occupational therapist
Physical therapist
Therapy aides
Social workers
Nurse
Pediatric neurologist
Pediatrician
Speech and hearing consultant
Psychologist

About 18 months ago one of the children was hospitalized for several weeks at a rehabilitation hospital that had a very aggressive nutritional program. We were amazed at how much weight he had gained while in the hospital. We had known that most of our children were considerably under the 3rd percentile in both height and weight, but had more or less accepted this as concomitant with their other profound handicaps. The fact that one of these children had gained weight while in the hospital made us feel uncomfortable in having largely neglected the nutritional aspects of our program. We had been pleased to see the progress made in other areas by a team of professionals who refused to accept the traditional custodial attitudes and programs for handicapped children, and who were very aggressive and imaginative in utilizing various therapies. We speculated that a similar aggressive approach concerning nutrition might further enhance the quality of life these children experience.

We decided that a nutritional survey of each child should be done to document his nutritional status. Table 8-3 is a summary of this nutritional assessment. Table 8-4 indicates the number of children having one or more substandard parameters.

Table 8-3
Nutritional Assessment of Children (n = 32) at EISEC

Parameter	% Below Normal
Squalene/wax ratio	60
Height for age	50
Weight for height	75
Skin-fold thickness	84
Midarm circumference	56
Midarm muscle circumference	41
Hematocrit	16

Table 8-4
Nutritional Index (n = 32)

No. Abnormal Parameters	No. Children
1	4
2	6
3	2
4	6
5	10
6	4
7	0

We also looked critically at each child and his family, and identified various factors that contributed to his undernutrition. Economic and social factors included:

1. Inadequate diet
   Poverty — 83% were on Medicaid
   Ignorance of nutrition
2. Excessive feeding time
3. Multiproblem families
4. Emotional atmosphere at meal times
   Anxiety
   Anger
   Frustration

Mechanical factors encountered included:

1. Spasticity (80%)
   Tongue thrust

       Bite reflex
       Inability to suck, chew, and swallow
       Inability to grasp and release
2. Athetosis
3. Flaccidity
4. Improper positioning
5. Poor hand-to-mouth coordination
6. Dependency on bottle
7. Poor dentition
8. Rumination

Some medical factors that interfered with feeding and nutrition, included:

1. Frequent infections
2. Overmedication of seizures
3. Undermedication of seizures
4. Constipation
5. Diarrhea or malabsorption
6. Poor energy level

The results of our nutrition project can be viewed from the effects it has had on specific children, and from the effects it has had on the program in general.

The boy whom I described initially lost most of the 12 lbs he had gained in the rehabilitation hospital when he returned home. One reason was the fatalistic attitude of his deeply religious parents, who said, "Whatever will be, will be." Another problem was that, when the orthopedist told his parents, "Gee, he looks good," in an effort to be supportive, the parents used this statement to justify their not being more aggressive in feeding their son. After this was discussed with the orthopedist he switched to, "Gee, he looks awful," and the parents made more effort to provide better food and increased feeding time.

Another girl 8-years-old, after a year's effort by the occupational therapist, teacher, and dietitian, moved from sucking a bottle of milk to learning to chew a rather thick paste of the family's meals prepared in a blender. She was also painstakingly taught to spoon-feed herself and is now 70% successful in doing so.

A third child was being underfed, eating only the daily hot lunch sent along with him by his grandmother. The staff was able to work sensitively with him, informing him about diet and nutrition, which enabled him to increase the quality, quantity, and variety of his meals, resulting in improvement of the child's nutrition.

These three children are representative of what can be done by a team approach directed at nutrition and feeding. The effects our nutritional survey had on the project in general were quite varied, and at times unexpected. We tried to correct those factors interfering with feeding and nutrition.

The occupational and physical therapists work with the teachers in positioning the children, utilizing special feeding tables and chairs that hold the child upright and support his head. They desensitize the overactive bite reflexes and tongue thrusts. Children on bottles are being taught to take solids. The social workers and nurse work with parents to secure better food and more variety. Those children with seizures have had serum levels of anticonvulsants ascertained and regulation of the medication adjusted. Iron was given to those with anemia. Nutritional supplements were added as necessary.

The school lunch and school breakfast programs were explored, as well as the Woman, Infant, and Children's (WIC) program. A group of less retarded children attending another program in our building was also assessed. Documentation of their poor nutritional status was an impetus for administrators to bring a school lunch program to the school. No one previously had taken the initiative to do this, even though these children had been eligible for one. Our survey served to heighten the awareness of nutrition among other professionals and administrators throughout the mental retardation center.

We sought funds from several state, federal, and private organizations for a dietitian for the program, as well as food and nutritional supplements for the children. We learned that no one was interested at the time in supporting a research project. School lunch programs are associated with surplus foods and some of this food is inappropriate for our children. Federal guidelines that determine eligibility give no recognition to the functional age of a child. Thus a 10-year-old handicapped child functioning at the level of 10 months cannot obtain the formula he needs from the WIC program because they do not service children over 5 years of age.

We were unable to get program eligibility from any federal or state agency. What special foods we were able to obtain was by tediously filling out cumbersome forms for each individual child, documenting his handicap by collecting previous hospital and medical records, etc.

In October we were able to testify in Boston before a committee from the Department of Agriculture concerned with Child Nutrition Programs they funded. The chairman told us after our presentation that his committee had not been aware of the special nutritional needs of handicapped children, and had not known of the obstacles encountered in dealing with the bureaucracy. He promised to see that special needs of the handicapped received high priority in future guidelines of Child Nutrition Programs.

We were very gratified by the parents' support of our nutritional assessment project. They expressed great interest in learning more about diets, money management in selecting foods, and in learning better feeding techniques.

A grant was written and funded by the Department of Education of Massachusetts to hire a nutritionist half-time to implement a service program for the coming year. The goals of this program are to improve the nutritional status of our children, utilizing the techniques described earlier. We want to increase family participation and knowledge of good nutritional practices and mechanical feeding techniques. We want to increase staff awareness of the specific nutritional needs of handicapped children. We will evaluate this program by a nutritional assessment every six months, using the seven parameters described earlier, as well as by interviewing staff and parents.

The implications for pediatricians, dietitians, and nutritionists are clear:

1. A steady population of multiply-handicapped infants and children will be maintained every year from premature births, congenital abnormalities, and survivors of respirators used in managing older children with severe infections and trauma.

2. Public Law 94-142 will accelerate the number of multiply-handicapped children residing in the community and decrease the number of those formerly referred to residential institutions. Giving parents a role in placement decisions will guarantee their involvement in monitoring programs. They will demand excellence of all professionals involved with their children. It is to be expected that the nutritional aspects discussed here will be one of their major concerns.

3. Pediatricians and dietitians must become aware of the special feeding problems of the mutliply-handicapped child. They will have to become members of the team managing such children and become familiar with the expertise each team member has to contribute to the habilitation of these children.

9 Impact of Nutrition on Immune Function

Joseph J. Vitale, ScD, MD

In the past few years a great deal of progress has been made by immunologists in elucidating the functions and interactions of the various cell types that protect the host from infectious agents. Also, progress has been made in our understanding of how various nutrients, and the quality and quantity of various dietary components, affect our immune system.

Immune Function

Immune function, however defined, has been shown to be adversely affected by every nutritional deficiency studied. Lipidemia and hypercholesterolemia have also been shown to compromise some component of this defense system. Since space limits the treatment of the possible roles that nutrients play in cell-mediated and humoral immunity, I will focus on the clinical importance of the relationship between nutrition and immune function. The immune system will be reviewed briefly, the role of specific nutrients in this system will be described, and nutritional management of the immunosuppressed patient will be discussed.

Immunity implies protection against foreign materials, including cancer cells, that can result in disease; it is concerned with very specific responses made by a host who is challenged by foreign substances called antigens or immunogens. Whereas an antigen may not necessarily elicit an immune response, an immunogen always does. Bacterial, viral, fungal, protozoan, other parasitic organisms, and foreign cells can act as antigens or immunogens. Immunity involves three major responses that are generally classified as: 1) cell-mediated immune response, the thymus-dependent system often referred to as delayed hypersensitivity; 2) humoral anitbody response; and 3) the nonspecific immunity response, which includes phagocytosis and macrophage-mediated cytotoxicity.[1]

Historical perspective The complexity of the immune system was perhaps first suggested by studies in chickens, which have two primary immune organs: the thymus and the bursa of Fabricius. These organs are similar, as both are lymphoid organs and are embryologically derived from the gastrointestinal epithelium. The cells they process are the small lymphocytes. Nevertheless, the thymus and bursa are involved in different immune responses. Removal of the thymus produces defects in cellular immunity. On the other hand, a serious deficiency in antibody formation with near-normal cell-mediated immunity ensues when the bursa has been removed from the chick embryo.

The equivalent of the bursa in humans and other mammals has not been defined clearly, although the consensus is that the hematopoietic tissue itself may provide the appropriate environment for the maturation of the cells concerned with antibody production (humoral immunity). There is evidence that a thymus hormone, thymosin, may act at distant sites (eg, bone marrow) on stem cells or uncommitted lymphocytes to effect differentiation into T cells. The skin, mucous membranes, the integrity of cell membranes and of parenchymal cells, and fixed and floating macrophages are all considered components of the body's defense. Indeed, the immune system is so multifaceted that a defect in one component may be compensated for by the action of another. Also, the immune response is probably exaggerated, so that a defect in the activity of some component does not leave the host unprotected against foreign pathogens.

Cell-mediated immunity Cell-mediated immunity (Figure 9-1) is an independent immune system mediated by a subset of lymphocytes called T cells. Before entering the lymphoid tissue or the blood, these cells undergo primary differentiation in the thymus, where their surfaces develop certain receptor sites that commit each cell to react with a single antigenic determinant. Therefore, when foreign materials (ie, bacteria or other antigens) enter the body, lymphocytes bearing the appropriate antigen receptor site will combine with them. It is this antigen-antibody interaction that initiates immunologic activation as well as the induction and amplification of the so-called immune response. When the antigen and lymphocyte come in contact, the lymphocyte "turns on" (ie, divides and differentiates), "turns off" (becomes specifically tolerant), or ignores the antigen. The nature of the response depends on many factors, including the concentration of the antigen and the complex interaction with other lymphocytes and macrophages.

Currently under consideration are at least three subsets of T cells, "killer" cells, "helper" cells, and "suppressor" cells. Killer cells can actually destroy other cells. The helper T cells can enhance B-cell responses in the humoral immune system. Suppressor cells may inhibit T-helper and B-cell responses.

Lymphokines   A T cell differentiates when it is exposed to an antigen. When a differentiated T cell is exposed to this particular antigen again, it secretes many soluble factors called lymphokines. Therefore, in addition to the direct actions of T cells, the lymphokines can act in a number of ways in participating in the cell-mediated immune response:

1. The lymphokines may cause the circulating macrophages to secrete various lysosomal enzymes, thus accelerating the phagocytosis of the foreign material.

2. The lymphokines may act as a macrophage migration-inhibitory factor to immobilize macrophages.

3. The lymphokines may be chemotactic factors that increase vascular

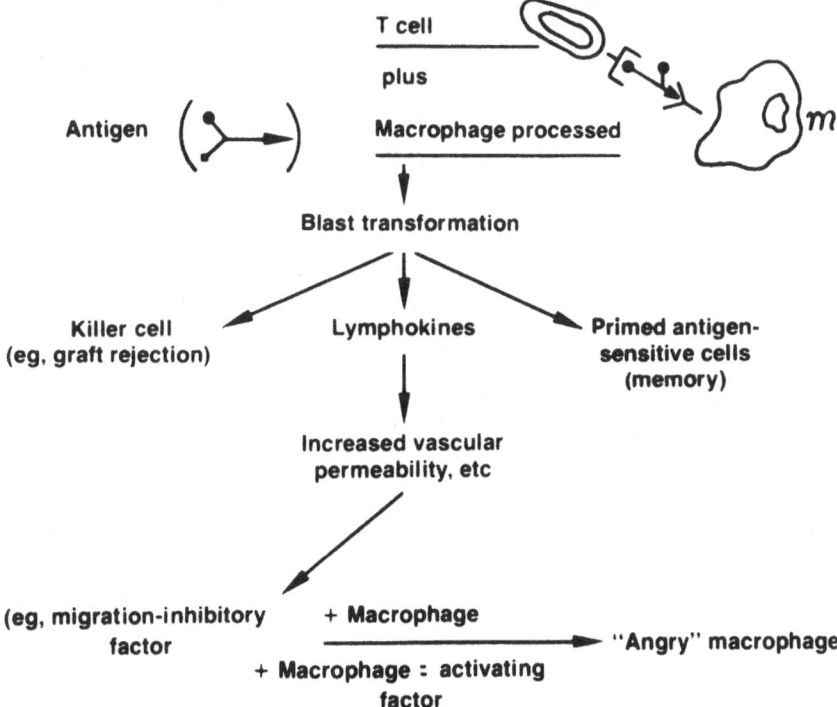

Figure 9-1 Cell types in cell-mediated immunity.

permeability, and therefore enhance cellular access of the macrophage to the site where the antigen and lymphocyte are interacting.

4. The lymphokines may be mitogenic factors or substances that can help "recruit" previously uncommitted lymphocytes to multiply and differentiate for participation in the immune response.

5. The lymphokines may make macrophages more metabolically active or "angry," and therefore more effective in degrading the phagocytosed bacteria.

6. The lymphokines may be cytotoxic and may directly kill target cellls.

7. The lymphokine may be a transfer factor, a low-molucular-weight substance (about 10,000 daltons) that can be isolated from sensitized cells and can transfer immunity to nonsensitized cells.

8. The lymphokine may be interferon, an antiviral agent that is species-specific, but nonspecific within one species. Interferons may be elaborated by the stimulated T cell and presumably may inhibit intracellular viral replication. (Evidence suggests that any cell, in response to viral infection, can synthesize an interferon-like substance.)

Unquestionably, lymphokines as well as T cells may cooperate with B cells; this cooperation may extend to macrophage intervention (see Figure 9-1). Mounting evidence indicates that macrophages may play a role in regulating T-cell and B-cell responsiveness. For T cells, macrophages appear to affect antigen recognition, ie, they may help to "process" the antigen for presentation to the T cell (see Figure 9-2). In the absence of the

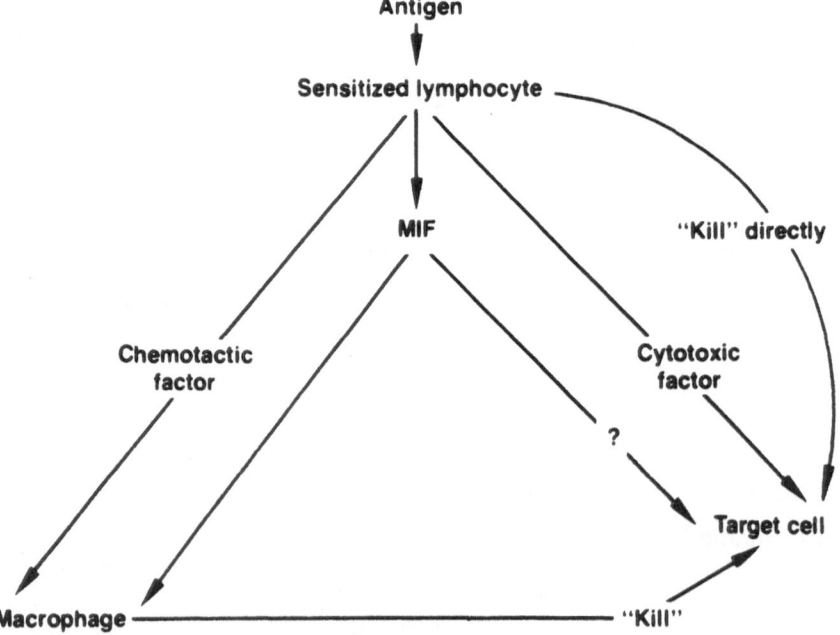

Figure 9-2 Pathways of delayed hypersensitivity.

macrophages, interaction of T cells and antigen may be absent or diminished. Another cell, called an M cell, has been suggested. It is neither a T or B cell and is marrow-dependent.

Humoral immunity   Humoral immunity involves B lymphocytes (B cells), which secrete antibodies by a complex differentiation pathway. The B cells have membrane-bound immunoglobulins (Ig) similar to those eventually secreted by the plasma cell. Unsensitized B cells do not elaborate Ig. Rather, when activated by antigen, B cells differentiate into Ig-secreting cells or plasma cells.

The antibodies comprise five Ig classes: IgM, IgG, IgE, IgD, and IgA. Each has a somewhat different function in the body. IgM occurs primarly in the blood stream and is probably the first antibody formed after an antigenic challenge. IgG, the predominant immunoglobulin in the blood and extracellular fluid, is the second antibody produced after antigenic challenge; it is the class of proteins responsible for the gamma-globulin band seen when serum is subjected to electrophoresis. IgE is the antibody responsible for allergic manifestations and for anaphylaxis. The function of IgD is not clearly understood at this time.

One of the first immunologic defenses that a foreign body or bacterium encounters while attempting to penetrate a mucous membrane, whether in the gastrointestinal tract, the pulmonary tree, or the genitourinary tract, is secretory immunoglobulin (S-IgA). This component of the immune system consists of two molecules of IgA (coupled by a joining of "J" chain) and one molecule of secretory piece. Secretory piece and IgA are made by different cells, and S-IgA can be secreted onto the surface of the mucous membrane because of its association with secretory piece. Thus, patients with defective production of S-IgA are highly susceptible to various infections and allergic responses of the lung and gut.

Complement   Once antibody is formed, it may protect the host by activating a series of complex enzymes that are collectively called complement. Complement is a complex of at least nine major protein components, with subsets or subunits of the major protein that have adherence as well as cytotoxic properties, and interact with the antibody-antigen complex to dispose of the antigen. The antibody molecule combines with antigen and this antibody-antigen complex binds with the first component of complement. A cascade of events follows that eventually leads to the release of a number of active proteins or kinins and various chemotactic factors. These interact with leukocytes that migrate to the site of the antigen-antibody complex, there to participate in, and enhance phagocytosis. Furthermore, as the events continue, seven to nine complement components elaborate proteolytic and lipolytic enzymes capable of destroying cell walls and membranes. Lysis and destruction of the antigen or bacteria result. Macrophages then engulf these destroyed cells. A variety of cells produce complement proteins, including intestinal mucosal cells and macrophages.

Additional T- and B-cell differences   Within peripheral lymphoid tissue, the T and B cells occupy defined regions. The B cells generally are found in the germinal centers and in the medullary cords of the lymphoid tissue, whereas the T cells occur in the deep cortical or paracortical areas. The defined receptor sites on B cells, as on T cells, can recognize distinct and separate antigens. On B cells, the receptors appear to be IgG and IgM molecules. The receptors on T cells are still under investigation, but under electrophoresis they appear to be immunoglobulin-like.

From a morphologic point of view, little or no difference exists between T and B lymphocytes, as evidenced by light or electron microscopy. However, T cells are distinguishable from B cells by a variety of surface markers and by their responsiveness to antigens. Certain antigens or mitogens are specific for T cells, eg, phytohemagglutinin (PHA) and concanavalin A (Con A), while others such as lipopolysaccharides are specific for B cells. The presence of immunoglobulins can be demonstrated rather easily on the surface of B cells, but not on T cells. Other evidence for the dichotomy of T and B cells comes from immunologically deficient patients. Patients with Bruton-type congenital agammaglobulinemia or B-cell deficiency cannot make antibodies but have near-normal cell-mediated immunity. On the other hand, patients with Di George's syndrome have a congenital absence of lymphocytes in the thymus, which results in T-cell deficiency and impaired cell-mediated immunity; however, these patients have near-normal amounts of humoral antibody. Additionally, the removal of the thymus from newborn mice renders them incapable of rejecting allogeneic skin grafts. This phenomenon was demonstrated in the nu/nu strain of mice, which have few, if any lymphocytes in their thymus glands.

Although immune and host defense systems appear to be distinct, they are nevertheless interrelated. For example, some antigens appear to be specific for B cells (eg, *Pseudomonas aeruginosa*). Yet, in patients with defective T-cell function, this gram-negative pathogen can produce disease. It is generally held that defective T-cell immunity is associated with infectious diseases caused by certain pathogenic bacteria, mycobacteria, viruses, fungi, and parasites, whereas B-cell deficiency may be associated with other types of bacterial infections (eg, those caused by diphtheria, tetanus, and pneumococcus) as well as with most viral infections. These distinctions may not be entirely valid. Indeed B cells, perhaps in a fashion similar to T suppressor cells, may elaborate "blocking" antibodies that "cover" the antigen, thus preventing interaction of T cell and antigen.

Nonspecific immunity   Included in the category of nonspecific immunity is phagocytosis, in which polymorphonuclear leukocytes and macrophages protect the host against invasion by various organisms. Lysozymes discharged from various granules within these cells and from complement are also involved in the killing of microorganisms. Nonspecific immunity might also include opsonins, which are probably antibodies. Furthermore, these plus other unidentified factors in serum cause the antigen to adhere to the phagocyte, facilitating phagocytosis.

The macrophages, essential components of humoral and cell-mediated immunity, are distinct from T or B cells and may be of the floating or fixed phagocytic types. The floating types include the polymorphonuclear leukocytes and monocytes in the blood. Fixed macrophages in tissue (histiocytes) include the Kupffer cells and the alveolar macrophages. Kupffer cells are found in the liver sinusoids, whereas the alveolar macrophages occur in the pulmonary alveolar septa and air spaces.

Macrophages may engulf cellular debris or may actually destroy cellular bacteria. In addition, T-cell lymphokines may activate other capacities of macrophages. This activity can lead to destruction of bacteria and cells, offshoots of which include production of hydrogen peroxide, free radical formation, and catheptic enzyme activity.

Tests for immune competency   Several tests to measure immune competency are easily done, whereas others require rather sophisticated laboratory facilities. For example, if a simple white blood cell count reveals leukopenia or is less than 1500/cu mm, some defect in immune responsiveness should be presumed.

The number of T or B cells in the blood can be determined by various techniques. The lymphocyte population consists of approximately 60% T cells, 20% B cells, and the rest uncommitted cells. These techniques, however, require more sophisticated laboratory facilities than are usually found in a physician's office.

Skin testing or a test for delayed hypersensitivity by the intradermal injection of an antigen, such as tuberculin, on the inner surface of the forearm, is informative. If, after 48 to 72 hours, an induration of 5 mm or more appears, a positive delayed hypersensitivity is present, and normal cellular immune function can be assumed if there was previous exposure to tuberculosis. For humoral immunity, other antigens can be administered to elicit anitbody response.

A test now used in many laboratories is the determination of T lymphocyte blast transformation. One can measure the response of lymphocytes to certain mitogens. The subsequent synthesis of DNA can be followed by incubating isolated lymphocytes with tritiated thymidine. Two mitogens commonly used for assessing T cells are Con A and PHA, whereas lipopolysaccharide is used to assess B-cell function. The amount of tritiated thymidine taken up provides some assessment of the immune system. The turned-on lymphocyte is rich in mitochondria and other cellular organelles.

Also useful is measurement of the response of the individual to active sensitization. Fourteen to twenty-one days after dinitrochlorobenzene

(DNCB) has been applied to the skin, a state of delayed sensitization is induced and can be demonstrated by a second application of DNCB to a different skin area. If cellular immunity is intact, an erythematous lesion and blistering are observed on the second challenge.

Testing for macrophage-inhibitory factors may be helpful, but this complicated procedure is available only in a research laboratory. Immune status can be ascertained, to some extent, from lymph node or rectal biopsies of bone marrow aspirates. These are certainly not used routinely, and they do involve a certain risk. Levels of immunoglobulins IgA, IgM, or IgG, and C3 complement component may indicate adequacy of immune competency. In the absence of T cells, B cells, or phagocytes, an individual is at great risk to all sorts of infection. Patients with complement deficiency are also particularly susceptible to infections. Individuals with immunodeficiency diseases usually die early as infants from overwhelming infection. Recently, researchers and clinicians have been exploring the role of immunocompetency in the development of cancer.

A patient's ability to mount an immune response has nutritional, environmental (eg, drug-related), and genetic determinants. For a discussion of environmental and genetic determinants, the reader is referred to *Harrison's Principles of Internal Medicine,*[2] a recent article by Cunningham,[3] and one by Kumar[4]. The major histocompatibility complex controlling various immune functions in humans is the HLA complex (HLA-A, HLA-B, HLA-C, and HLA-D) on chromosome 6. This complex probably corresponds to the murine counterpart, serologically defined as the H-2 locus on chromosome 17. This locus (H-2K and H-2D) can be fragmented into subsections or regions that are separable by genetic recombinations (ie, by chromosomal crossover among subregions.) It has been demonstrated that certain regions have genes controlling: 1) T-cell regulation of antibody formation to thymus-dependent antigens (in the immunoresponsive region); 2) the levels of several components of the complement system; 3) resistance to bone marrow transplantation; and 4) graft rejection. Other immunologic functions can also be demonstrated on the H-2 locus.

Clearly, immunosuppression is a desired effect only in special cases, as in the patient who has received an organ transplant, and in whom immunosuppressive drugs may be used to inhibit graft rejection. (Interestingly, some investigators are beginning to study the effects of specific nutrient deficiencies or special diets that may cause immunosuppression, as adjuvants to immunosuppressive drug therapy.)

NUTRITION AND IMMUNITY

Any nutrient excess or deficiency that adversely affects any of the complement components or the maturation of T cells or B cells, or that inhibits DNA synthesis, cell division, or replication would be expected to affect cell-mediated immunity and humoral immunity responses, and could place the individual at risk to infection. Macrophages also require a certain amount of energy to release their proteolytic and lipolytic enzymes for the destruction of bacterial cells. Any nutrient involved in these biochemical reactions, if deficient, would also be expected to render the cell immunoincompetent.

People who are malnourished are more susceptible to infectious diseases and, in such individuals, the disease may run a more severe course. For example, measles is usually mild in the well-nourished individual and can be deadly in the malnourished one. Moreover, infections from any cause (viral, bacterial, or fungal) precipitate a catabolic response resulting in negative nitrogen balance, possible tissue pathology, and consequently a further compromise of nutritional status that renders the host even more susceptible to infectious agents.

Effects of Specific Nutrients on Immunity

Not every cell or organ is affected equally by a given nutrient deficiency. For example, folic acid deficiency would be expected to affect the more rapidly dividing cells since a major biochemical function of the vitamin is related to DNA and RNA synthesis. Thus, with folic acid deficiency one would expect to see biochemical and morphologic changes in the white cells of the gastrointestinal tract. Some white cell types are being synthesized every few hours to days, the villous epithelial cells of the small bowel replace themselves completely every 2 or 3 days, and the red cell has a life span of 120 days. Thus, the requirement for folate is high for normal leukopoiesis and hematopoiesis and for regeneration of crypt cells (progenitors of the epithelial cells of the villi).

Hepatic cells, on the other hand, have a very slow turnover rate. Thus, the liver is not as susceptible to the initial effects of folate deficiency, nor would it be the first organ to show signs or symptoms of folate deficiency. If folate deficiency is chronic, then anemia, infection, and malabsorption would result in a worsening of the nutritional state and would eventually affect other organs, including the liver. However, folate deficiency is induced in the patient with liver disease, since the liver is a major site for the conversion of dietary absorbed folate to coenzyme forms.

Regardless of the etiology of the malnourished state (eg, protein deficiency, liver disease, malabsorption), immunocompetency and, particularly, cell-mediated responses can be hindered.

Calories No evidence indicates that, within reason, caloric restriction has any impact on immune function as long as nutrient intake is adequate. Indeed, caloric restriction throughout life may be beneficial: animals fed adequate but restricted diets (in terms of calories) live 30% to 40% longer, their optimum immune function peaks later, and they have fewer spontaneous tumors than animals that are fed ad libitum.[5,7] Certainly, obese patients are at greater risk to a number of diseases and to decreased longevity. Infections that lead to catabolic responses[8] resulting in a rapid weight loss, in negative nitrogen balance, and in loss of essential nutrients, often result in induced deficiency states in the severely calorie-restricted or marasmic individual. Such an individual would undoubtedly be rendered immunosuppressed.[9]

Protein Protein nutriture may markedly influence immune function. However, "pure" protein deficiency occurs rarely. The patient who comes closest to having a pure protein deficiency is the child with cystic fibrosis who presents with several of the signs and symptoms of kwashiorkor. To label the child with cystic fibrosis or with kwashiorkor as "protein-calorie" malnourished, however, would not only be naive but sophistic. The designation of protein-calorie malnutrition in association with immune function is too often used carelessly. The clinical picture in these patients is much more complex than is commonly recognized.

In recent years, many immunologic studies have been conducted not only on patients with the kwashiorkor-like syndrome, but also on those with clinical disorders associated with varying degrees of malnutrition. For example, the person with chronic alcoholism who is admitted to the hospital for the fourth time with the diagnosis of chronic pancreatitis usually presents with iron, folate, protein, pyridoxine, and vitamin A deficiency signs and symptoms, as well as osteomalacia (vitamin D deficiency) and hypoalbuminemia. The patient also has some liver dysfunction and thus cannot convert some of the ingested nutrients into their active coenzyme forms (eg, vitamin D into 25-hydroxycholecalciferol). Although the patient may have been ingesting the required amounts of the nutrients, a diseased organ may prevent their absorption or use. The deficiency that results when a disorder within the body interferes with the ability to use a dietary nutrient is known as a secondary or induced deficiency. In contrast, an individual who is not ingesting the required amounts of a nutrient has a primary deficiency. Alcoholic patients usually present with both primary and secondary deficiencies. As a result of pancreatitis, these patients probably have moderate to severe malabsorption. Such patients may also be anergic by skin testing, and their T cells may respond poorly to stimulation by mitogens. To say that malnutrition is the cause of this anergy would be correct, but to imply, as many published articles seem to, that it is due to protein and/or calorie deficiency would be misleading and inaccurate. Nonetheless, individuals with hypoalbuminemia from any cause are usually immunosuppressed. Surprisingly, though, animal studies suggest that long-term diets providing marginal protein levels are associated with enhanced immunocompetency.[10]

Children or adults with mild to moderate hypoalbuminemia (less than 3 g/100 ml) may present with defects in cellular and humoral immunity, delayed killing of phagocytosed antigens, and defects in tissue integrity (eg, atrophy of the thymus and gut epithelial tissue.)[11-13] Delayed hypersensitivity is absent and leukopenia is evident (T-cell numbers are depressed). However, T-cell blast transformation may be normal in these patients. The reason for a normal finding in such a situation is understandable. The test calls for only a limited number of cells, whereas the patient requires a critical mass of immune cells to combat the infectious agent.

Children with what is often thought to be kwashiorkor present with a clinical syndrome that has signs and symptoms of several essential nutritional deficiencies together with an infection. What nutritional signs and symptoms are present depends on the patient's prior nutritional status and on the type of infection to which he or she succumbs. Conversely, it may be shown that, depending on the most limiting nutrient, one might be able to predict the type of infecting agent. For example, complement deficiency is usually associated with pneumococcal infections, and magnesium deficiency renders the host deficient in complement activation. It is of interest that chronic alcoholics usually have pneumococcal infections and an associated magnesium deficiency. Epidemiologic studies suggest that the clinical picture of kwashiorkor itself is usually precipitated by an infectious process in the already nutritionally compromised marasmic child, thus activating the vicious cycle of infection and malnutrition. An immunologically healthy child who develops a viral gastroenteritis will suffer only minimal consequences. In the somewhat marasmic child whose nutritional reserves are depleted, a mild viral infection may precipitate respiratory infection, diarrhea, and hypoalbuminemia, as well as signs and symptoms of deficiency of one or more of the essential nutrients.

Children with hypoalbuminemia or kwashiorkor, or adults with associated protein malnutrition, usually have normal or high levels of immunoglobulins. Indeed, the abundance of plasma cells in various tissues suggests that the patient is attempting to mount an appropriate immune response.[14,15] Some studies suggest, however, that these patients are unable to exhibit a normal antibody response to some antigens.[16] With decreased numbers of T cells (leukopenia) and therefore, perhaps, decreased T helper cells, the response of the B cells to an antigen may be meager, with resultant decreased antibody production.

Results of studies of antibody response to antigens in malnourished patients may vary for three reasons. First, the antigens used may not be standardized or specified. Second, certain antigens, such as measles or polio, differ from other bacterial toxoids in the way they affect B cells or involve T helper or T suppressor cells. For example, some antigens depend primarily on B cells for antibody production, whereas other antigens require T helper function. Third, blood complement components or macrophages amplify the biologic effects of antibodies. Knowledge of the status of these components in the subject is necessary before ineffective antibody production can be implicated with certainty in protein and/or calorie deficiency.

There is no clear indication that the ability either to phagocytose or to kill bacteria is seriously impaired in the patient with hypoalbuminemia. Kinetic studies show that the rate of killing seems to be delayed, but eventually the bacteria engulfed seem to be killed. Again, one should remember that although all bacteria in the test tube are killed eventually, the patient is probably still at risk with defective killing. The delay in killing may be related to deficiencies of essential nutrients other than protein. Phagocytosis and killing depend on energy, and the enzyme systems involved in effective killing include iron, iodine, pyridoxine, and folic acid.

In summary, protein deficiency (hypoalbuminemia), however induced, results in generalized hypoplasia leading to depressed bone marrow activity, decreased numbers of stem cells able to differentiate into T cells and B cells, and atrophy of lymphoid organs, mucous membranes, and the gastrointestinal tract. This series of events places the subject at high risk for developing infection.

Iron   Iron-deficiency anemia is considered the cardinal nutritional problem in the world. It is difficult, at times, to remember that iron deficiency can exist without anemia or that depletion of iron stores without any change in blood values can be associated with defects in DNA synthesis and in cell proliferation, with tissue changes, and with enzyme aberrations. Any one or all three of these defects or changes may affect immune status. Iron deficiency, even of the mild type and without anemia, may render the phagocyte incompetent.[17,18] Myeloperoxidase, an enzyme in the macrophage required for killing, is iron-dependent and is depressed by a deficiency of iron. Indeed, the first sign of iron deficiency is not seen in the red cell but rather in a white cell, the polymorphonuclear leukocyte. Iron deficiency probably affects all microphages and macrophages, both fixed and floating, thereby reducing their ability to kill ingested bacteria.[19] Iron deficiency also affects folate utilization.[20] As mentioned earlier, folic acid is required for DNA and RNA synthesis, and therefore secondary folate deficiency may play a significant role in immunosuppression in iron-deficient persons.

Experiments with patients with chronic mucocutaneous candidiasis, a fungal disease, have indicated that the abnormal immunologic status of these patients can be linked to disturbances in their iron metabolism.[21] Joynson et al[22] have shown that iron deficiency depresses the incorporation of tritiated thymidine into the DNA of human proliferating lymphocytes. In other studies using HeLa cells, it was noted that, during mitosis, iron present in the nucleolus is normally transferred to the chromosomes, but when the iron-chelating agent, deferoxamine, is introduced to the culture of the living cells, DNA synthesis is inhibited.[23] The same defect in normal synthesis is found in patients with iron-deficiency anemia.[24] In our own earlier studies with protein-calorie–deficient children, host defense mechanisms were affected not by the status of iron nutriture at any given moment, but rather by shifts in iron metabolism.[18]

Vitamin A   More recently, vitamin A has been shown to play some role in cellular immunity. Cortisone or steroids suppress immune responsiveness. The administration of vitamin A to cortisone-treated animals appears to abolish the immunosuppressive effects of cortisone.[25] The mechanism involved is not clear although vitamin A administration may protect by stabilizing lysosomal membranes of immune cells. Vitamin A deficiency also results in epithelial tissue changes (eg, gastrointestinal and tracheal tissues) resulting in a decreased "barrier" system to ever-present pathogens. Vitamin A deficiency has also been shown to affect adversely T-cell blast transformation and antibody production in animals.[26]

Polyunsaturated fatty acids   In several studies,[27-29] the administration of polyunsaturated fatty acids (PUFA) in relatively high concentrations results in the depression of T-cell function. Animals lost their ability to reject skin allografts when fed diets high in PUFA.[26] PUFA have also been used as an adjuvant to immunosuppression in renal transplant patients.[28] Animals fed diets high in PUFA have diminished T-cell responses to mitogen.[29] The mechanism by which PUFA affect immune functions is not clear. More recently, several studies have shown that hyperlipidemia and particularly hypercholesterolemia are associated with depressed cellular and humoral responses.[30] While patients with hypercholesterolemia may be more susceptible to cardiovascular disease, they appear to be less susceptible to neoplasia. This may not be true for "normocholesterolemic" individuals. There is sufficient evidence to suggest that PUFA are not only immunosuppressive but are promoters of oncogenesis as well, since feeding diets high in polyunsaturated fatty acids, which will lower serum cholesterol levels, may be associated with an increased risk to neoplasia.[29] Indeed, a recent study suggests that lowering serum cholesterol levels in normal subjects may result in an increased incidence of colon cancer.[31]

Nutritional Management

All patients require nutritional support. The critical question, of course, is how to provide it. In the patient who is receiving total parenteral nutrition, attention must be paid to the increased requirements for most essential nutrients. Not long ago patients receiving all nutrients via the intravenous route developed deficiencies of essential fatty acids, copper, or zinc. Any one of these deficiencies affects immune competency, but at the time physicians puzzled about why these patients were not progressing well.

An analogous situation occurs in the child who is recovering from protein-calorie malnutrition and who is undergoing a rapid rate of "catch-up" growth. Unless this child is also given adequate levels of essential nutrients, deficiency states may be induced. There is much to be learned about the qualitative aspects of the diet for the sick patient, beyond replacing missing nutrients and correcting nutritional deficits. For example, it has been taught that protein intake should be kept at a minimum in the patient with hepatic encephalopathy to minimize blood ammonia levels. Recent evidence suggests that the administration of protein in the form of an amino acid mixture (which is different from what is considered an ideal mixture) mitigates the coma usually associated with severe liver disease.[31]

And so it may be with a number of diseases. Optimal nutritional support may mean rather significant deviations from what we now consider to be ideal nutrition. This is particularly true in cancer patients who may already be immunosuppressed as a result of their tumors (which may be immunosuppressive) or chemotherapy (immunosuppressive drugs.) It should be stressed that depressed cellular immunity and oncogenesis may not be causally related. However, most health professionals agree that, for the hospitalized patient, use of any dietary regimen that depresses immune function is not prudent.

Although every known nutrient studied has some effect on immune function, until now only deficiency states have been shown to depress immune function. An excellent review on the effects of single nutrient deficiencies on immunologic functions has been published recently.[33] However, adequate diets, depending on the qualitative composition or the amount fed, may suppress immune function. For example, diets high in PUFA can be immunosuppressive[27,28]; rapid rates of growth, rather than slow rates of growth, are associated with a more rapid decline in immune function[5-7]; and, in mice, low-protein (but not protein-deficient) diets are immunostimulatory whereas high-protein diets are immunosuppressive.[10] These and other observations suggest that further studies will be needed to determine the possible benefits or risks to cancer patients (or any other debilitated patients) in "force-feeding" them diets containing unusually low or high quantities of any nutrient. Thus, rapid recovery from weight loss, rapid weight gain, or ingestion of high-protein diets may conceivably be detrimental to the patient with cancer or any other debility.

Specific nutrients may be more essential for the multiplication of pathogenic organisms of even preneoplastic or allogeneic cells than for the maintenance of the host. Thus, as suggested by Murray et al,[34] starvation may actually suppress disease, and feeding may exacerbate the disease process. Furthermore, the clinical counterpart of starvation, anorexia nervosa, is not associated with an increased risk to infection. Situations may also arise in which feeding diets low or deficient in specific nutrients may have beneficial consequences. For example, iron deficiency with or without anemia can enhance the proliferation of syngeneic grafted bone-marrow transplants in lethally irradiated rats.[35] Futhermore, the administration of a preparation of PUFA to humans with cadaveric renal transplants can improve graft survival time.[28] An iron-deficient preparation or an induced mild iron deficiency coupled with a low-fat, high-protein diet may someday prove useful in hematopoietic or organ transplantation or in cancer patients. Obviously, we are at the frontier of understanding of the complex interactions among nutrients, immunocompetency, and host defense systems.

CONCLUSIONS

Almost any nutritional deficiency, however induced, if severe enough and of chronic duration, might affect some component of the host defense system, including the various cell types and tissues. The skin and mucous membranes are effective barriers to the penetration of bacterial agents, and any nutritional deficiency that affects these tissues would compromise resistance to penetration by organisms. Certain nutrient excesses, deficiencies, or imbalances adversely affect the complement components, the maturation of T cells and B cells, DNA synthesis, cell division, and replication. Such situations would be expected to affect cell-mediated immunity and humoral immunity responses and could place the individual at risk for infection.

It must be stressed, however, that cellular or humoral immune responses may normally be exaggerated and that some decrease in either component in an in vitro or in vivo test system does not necessarily mean that the individual is immunologically compromised. Furthermore, the host's defense system is multifaceted and a defect in one component may be compensated for by activation of other components in the same system.

REFERENCES

1. Roitt IM; *Essential Immunology,* London, Blackwell Scientific Publications, 1977.
2. Thorn GW (ed): *Harrison's Principles of Internal Medicine*, ed 8, New York, McGraw-Hill Book Co Inc, 1977.
3. Cunningham BA: The structure and function of histocompatibility antigens. *Sci Am* 237:96, 1977.
4. Kumar V: Diseases of immunity: basic immunology, in Robbins SL, Cotran R (eds): *Pathologic Basis of Disease*. Philadelphia, WB Saunders Co, 1979, pp 262–278.
5. Yunis EJ, Greenberg LJ: Immunopathology of aging. *Fed Proc* 33:2017, 1974.

6. McCay CM, Crowell MF, Maynard LA: The effect of retarded growth upon the length of life span and upon the ultimate body size. *J Nutr* 10:63–79, 1935.

7. Stutman O: Cell-mediated immunity and aging. *Fed Proc* 33:2028, 1974.

8. Beisel WR: Magnitude of the host nutritional responses to infection. *Am J Clin Nutr* 30: 1236, 1977.

9. Vitale JJ: Impact of nutrition on vitamin metabolism: an unexplored area. *Am J Clin Nutr* 30: 1473, 1977.

10. Cooper WC, Good RA, Mariani R: Effect of protein insufficiency on immune responsiveness. *Am J Clin Nutr* 27: 647, 1974.

11. Smythe PM, Brereton-Stiles GG, Grace HJ, et al: Thymolymphatic deficiency and depression of cell-mediated immunity in protein-calorie malnutrition. *Lancet* 2: 939–943, 1971.

12. Sellmeyer E, Bhettay E, Truswell AS, et al: Lymphocyte transformation in malnourished children. *Arch Dis Child* 47: 429–435, 1972.

13. Faulk WP, Vitale JJ: Immunology, in Schneider HA, Anderson CE, Coursin DB (eds): *Nutritional Support of Medical Practice.* New York, Harper & Row Publishers Inc, 1977, pp 341–346.

14. Munson D, Franco D, Arbeter A, et al: Serum levels of immunoglobulins, cell-mediated immunity and phagocytosis in protein-calorie malnutrition. *Am J Clin Nutr* 27: 625, 1974.

15. Alvarado J, Luthringer DG: Serum immunoglobulins in edematous protein-calorie malnutrition. *Clin Pediatr* 10: 174, 1971.

16. Law DK, Dudrick SJ, Abdou NI: Immunocompetence of patients with protein-calorie malnutrition. The effects of nutritional repletion *Ann Intern Med* 79: 545–550, 1973.

17. MacDougall LG, Anderson R, Katz J: The immune response in iron-deficient children: impaired cellular defense mechanisms with altered humoral components. *J Pediatr* 86: 833–843, 1975.

18. Arbeter A, Echeverri L, Franco D, et al: Nutrition and infection. *Fed Proc* 30: 1421–1428, 1971.

19. Baggs RB, Miller SA: Defect in resistance to *Salmonella typhomurium* in iron-deficient rats. *J Infect Dis* 130: 409, 1974.

20. Velez H, Restrepo A, Vitale JJ, et al: Folic acid deficiency secondary to iron deficiency in man. *Am J Clin Nutr* 19: 27–36, 1966.

21. Higgs JM, Wells, RS: Chronic muco-cutaneous candidiasis: associated abnormalities of iron metabolism. *Br J Dermatol* 86: 88, 1977.

22. Joynson DHM, Walker DM, Jacobs A, et al: Defect of cell-mediated immunity in patients with iron-deficiency anemia. *Lancet* 2: 1058–1059, 1972.

23. Robbins E, Pederson T: Iron deficiency and cell-mediated immunity: defects in DNA synthesis. *Proc Natl Acad Sci USA* 66: 1244, 1970.

24. Hershko C, Karsai A, Eylon L, et al: The effect of chronic iron deficiency on some biochemical function of the hemopoietic tissue. *Blood* 36: 321–329, 1970.

25. Cohen BE, Cohen IK: Vitamin A: adjuvant and steroid antagonist in the immune response. *J Immunol* 3: 1376, 1973.

26. Rogers AE, Herndon BJ, Newberne PM: Induction by dimethyhydrazine of intestinal carcinoma in normal rats fed high or low levels of vitamin A. *Cancer Res* 33: 1003–1009, 1973.

27. Mertin J, Hunt R: Influence of polyunsaturated fatty acids on survival of skin allografts and tumor incidence in mice, *Proc Natl Acad Sci USA* 73:928, 1976.

28. McHugh MI, Wilkinson R, Elliott RW, et al: Immunosuppression with polyunsaturated fatty acids in renal transplantation. *Transplantation* 24: 263–267, 1977.

29. Broitman SA, Vitale JJ, Vavrousek-Jakuba E, et al: Polyunsaturated fat, cholesterol and large bowel tumorigenesis. *Cancer Res* 40:2455, 1977.

30. Kos WL, Loria RM, Snodgrass MJ, et al: Inhibition of host resistance by nutritional hypercholesterolemia. *Infect Immun* 26:658, 1979.

31. Williams RR, Sorlie PD, Feinlieb M, et al: Cancer incidence by levels of cholesterol. *JAMA* 245: 247-252, 1981.

32. Aquirre A, Funovics J, Wescorp RIC, et al: Parenteral nutrition in hepatic failure, in Fischer JE (ed): *Total Parenteral Nutrition*, Boston, Little Brown & Company, 1976, p 219.

33. Beisel WR, Edelman R, Nauss K, et al: Single-nutrient effects on immunologic function. *JAMA* 245: 53-58, 1981.

34. Murray J, Murray A, Murray M, et al: The biological suppression of malaria: an ecological and nutritional interrelationship of a host and two parasites. *Am J Clin Nutr* 31:1363-1366, 1978.

35. Rodday P, Bennett M, Vitale JJ: Delayed erythropoiesis in irradiated rats grafted with syngeneic marrow: effects of cytotoxic drugs and iron deficiency anemia. *Blood* 48:435, 1976.

10 The Effect of Infection on Host Nutritional Status

William R. Beisel, MD

Human beings generally experience a large number of infectious illnesses during their lifetime. Whether mild and self-limited, or of overwhelming severity, generalized infectious illnesses are all accompanied by transient derangements in the nutritional status of the host.[1,2] Thus, acute infectious illnesses constitute the most common transient threat to the nutritional status of normal persons. Some impact on host nutrition can be detected during infections with every variety of pathogenic microorganism studied; nutritional changes occur no matter whether a patient is well-nourished or poorly nourished at the time an infectious process begins.

Although infectious illnesses are the most common cause of transient impairments of host nutritional status, the patterns of response observed during an acute infectious illness are quite similar in many respects to those encountered during other acute inflammatory disease processes or after trauma.[3] Because infectious illnesses complicate other medical and surgical disease processes, the nutritional consequences of infection should be appreciated and understood by practitioners in every specialty so that supportive therapy can be utilized most effectively.

CATEGORIES OF NUTRIENT LOSS

The major effects of an infectious illness on nutritional status can be conceptualized as causing a loss or wastage of body nutrients.[1-3] In attempting to recognize and treat the nutritional consequences of an infection, the patterns of wastage can be categorized into two major classes. These are outlined in Table 10-1. Infection-induced wastages result from a combination of both absolute and functional losses of essential body nutrients. Each form of loss has relatively predictable patterns of onset and severity. Since the probable progression and magnitude of nutrient losses can be predicted to some degree, this information can, in turn, be used as a guide when planning supportive therapy for a patient.

Table 10-1
Forms of Infection-Induced Nutrient Loss

Absolute Losses

Measurable excretory losses of constituent nutrients from body tissues

Functional Losses

Losses occurring within body tissues due to metabolic or pathophysiologic responses

Overutilization of nutrients
Diversion of nutrients
Sequestration of nutrients

Absolute Losses

Absolute losses can be defined as measurable decreases in body nutrients that occur whenever an element is excreted or lost in amounts that are greater than its intake. These decreases have been measured conventionally for research purposes by performing metabolic balance studies.[2] Total protein deficits can also be estimated clinically by a fall in body weight, a reduction in muscle mass and skin-fold thickness, or by declining concentrations of serum albumin or transferrin. During an infectious process, absolute losses from the body begin shortly after the onset of fever and continue throughout the period of acute illness. The negative body balances represent the algebraic summation of all metabolic processes that participate in host defense responses. These responses include both anabolic processes and catabolic ones, with the latter predominating to cause the absolute deficits characteristic of febrile illnesses. The magnitude of these deficits is roughly proportional to the severity of the illness.[2]

Absolute losses from the body are typified by the decline in body nitrogen content that results from the combined effects of a diminished intake of food, the hypermetabolic effects of fever or other consequences of the infectious process per se, and an increased excretory loss of nitrogen via the urine, and in some instances, also via sweat and feces.

Wastage of body nitrogen serves as the prototype for absolute losses of other intracellular elements such as potassium, magnesium, phosphate, sulfur, and zinc. Absolute decreases of these individual elements are roughly proportional to the decreases of body weight experienced by patients with febrile illnesses. Some of this wastage can be reduced even during the infectious process by controlling fever and by increasing the intake of calories, proteins, and other nutrients. If absolute nutritional losses cannot be controlled during the acute phase of illness, they should be replaced promptly through the use of extra feeding during early convalescence.

Functional Losses

The second broad category of nutrient loss seen during an infectious process includes several functional changes that result from altered metabolic processes within body tissues. These functional losses can be considered to represent physiologic readjustments of the molecular mechanisms and metabolic pathways within body cells that alter patterns of nutrient utilization in response to the infectious process. These functional or physiologic responses can, or course, ultimately lead to absolute losses of body constituents.

The functional forms of wastage can be subdivided into three categories: (1) overutilization, (2) diversion, and (3) sequestration of essential body nutrients. Although these forms of functional wastage have been investigated in greatest detail through studies in experimental animals, their occurrence can also be documented by clinical studies performed in man.

Overutilization of nutrients   Acute infectious illnesses cause the body to accelerate or activate many normal intracellular physiologic and metabolic processes. As a result, the utilization of body nutrients is also accelerated and increased. The occurrence of fever and the initiation of other specific and nonspecific host defensive responses during an infectious process place increased demands on the normal body pools or storage depots for available nutrients. In the absence of an increased intake of these nutrients, body stores will become depleted.

An increase in body temperature causes a general speedup in the metabolic activity of body cells. It has been estimated that metabolic rates increase approximately 7% above basal for each degree Fahrenheit of body temperature elevation. This increased demand for body nutrients occurs despite the fact that sick patients lose their appetites and generally consume far smaller total quantities of nutrients than they do when they are healthy. To magnify the problem still further, the overutilization of nutrients during infection occurs in a manner that seems wasteful.

The most clearly defined example of overutilization of body nutrients involves the increased catabolism of various amino acids. Because of the need to synthesize increased amounts of carbohydrates to meet the caloric demands of fever, increased quantities of amino acids are used as substrates. These amino acids are deaminated, and their carbon skeletons are used to manufacture glucose. In this regard, the body seems willing to sacrifice contractile muscle protein in order to provide amino acids for use in the hepatic synthesis of glucose.[4] In less teleologic terms, muscle wastage occurs whenever the rates of degradation of muscle and structural body proteins exceed the ongoing or slowed rates of protein formation. Thus, when protein catabolism exceeds anabolism, free amino acids are liberated in excess quantities. These traverse the plasma pool to enter the liver, where they are used for several purposes.

Accelerated rates of gluconeogenesis during infections are due to the interplay of various carbohydrate-regulating hormones.[5] Because glucose production can be stimulated quickly by hormonal and enzyme responses, plasma amino acids are taken up by the liver and metabolized in excessive quantities. As an additional factor, body tissues possess only a sluggish adaptive ability to increase their utilization of fat depot lipids for fuel, especially during periods of stress. This combination of metabolic factors makes it difficult for the body to utilize its fat stores rapidly enough or in sufficient quantities to provide for the immediate caloric energy needed to meet the acute stressful conditions of infection. Further, the formation of ketone bodies as a possible source of cellular energy is minimized during infection by higher-than-normal insulin values.

Normally, during starvation, insulin levels are reduced and minimal protein catabolism occurs as a result of diminished cortisol levels. Thus, fat is burned as the major source of fuel. With acute stress, or infection or trauma, catecholamines are elevated as is cortisol; the former decreasing the utilization of insulin and the latter overriding the anabolic effects of insulin and increasing protein breakdown. A more judicious approach to the nutritional support of the patient probably necessitates knowing the levels of these hormones. In some cases, protein (or amino acids) with glucose and insulin may be required to override the catabolic effects of cortisol and catecholamines, whereas in the patient utilizing his fat stores, in the patient with a ketotic response, one may wish not to intervene except with protein.[6,7]

A second example of nutrient overutilization is shown by the observation that severe infectious illnesses may precipitate overt clinical deficiency states of several different vitamins.[8]

Diversion of nutrients   The second form of functional wastage is characterized by a diversion of nutrients into metabolic pathways that are less fully utilized during periods of normal health. Such a diversion of nutrients may have specific purposes for protecting the host. Such examples include the de novo synthesis of phagocytic cells, interferon, or specific antibody proteins.

As stated earlier, the infectious process also stimulates a marked acceleration in the uptake of plasma amino acids by the liver. Although some of these amino acids serve primarily to increase gluconeogenesis, many other amino acids that move into the liver are rapidly incorporated into hepatic enzymes or into newly synthesized acute-phase reactant plasma proteins.[9,10] This latter group of proteins includes haptoglobin, α-1-antitrypsin, α-2-macroglobulin, C-reactive protein, ceruloplasmin, and others. These acute-phase reactants are all glycoproteins that require carbohydrate components for their synthesis. Thus, accelerated glycoprotein synthesis also serves to divert both amino acids and carbohydrate moieties away from their calorigenic functions and into the structure of newly synthesized plasma proteins, whose specific function during inflammatory or infectious conditions remains largely unknown.

Other amino acids are diverted in excess into specific metabolic pathways. For example, tryptophan enters the kynurenine pathway during infectious illnesses in unusually large amounts.[11] This diversion of tryptophan leads to the formation and urinary excretion of unusually large quantities of kynurenine-pathway metabolites in the form of diazo reactants. Other portions of the available tryptophan pool appear to be diverted to form serotonin.

Sequestration of nutrients The third form of functional loss of nutrients occurs because of their sequestration within body pools or depots. Functional sequestration renders a nutrient essentially unavailable for its normal metabolic or physiologic purposes. As an example of this, sodium can become sequestered within body cells during periods of severe infectious illnesses, especially those accompanied by uncompensated acidosis. The sequestration of sodium in the intracellular space during infection is accompanied by hyponatremia of extracellular body fluids, and often by an inappropriate secretion of antidiuretic hormone. A patient with this derangement of salt and water metabolism is extremely susceptible to fluid overloading, and must be managed by carefully restricting the intake of fluids.

Another common form of sequestration during acute infection is the movement of iron into storage granules within cells of the liver, spleen, and bone marrow.[12] The stored iron appears to become functionally unavailable for use in red blood cell production as long as the infectious process persists. This sequestration in chronic infection may lead to the so-called anemia of infection. This sequestration of iron may have a purposeful role in host defense, however, for it has been shown that this iron is also rendered unavailable for use by bacteria that must acquire this essential nutrient to permit their proliferation.[13]

CONCLUSIONS

Because nutritional responses occur as a component feature of generalized infectious processes, it is important that practitioners in every specialty area anticipate the nutritional impact of an infectious illness and take proper supportive measures to reduce these effects. These supportive measures should be used to supplement the primary effects of specific antimicrobial therapy. For most patients, important aspects of nutritional therapy will include measures to ensure a continued intake of adequate quantities of protein precursors and sufficient calories to meet the basal needs of the patient, as well as the exaggerated needs that result from fever. Measures taken to control the febrile process will reduce nutritional wastages and thereby reduce total requirements for nutrients. In addition, an adequate vitamin intake should be assured.

On the other hand, depressed serum iron values and anemia will not respond to iron therapy as long as the infectious process persists. The corrections of hypoferremia can be accomplished only by eliminating or controlling the virulent invading microorganisms.

Finally, it must be emphasized that the nutritional deficits that accompany an infectious illness can increase patient susceptibility to subsequent, secondary, or superimposed infections.[14] Early convalescence remains a danger period, and nutritional therapy should be continued to prevent malnutrition and recurrent infections from developing into a vicious cycle.

REFERENCES

1. Beisel WR: Nutrient wastage during infection. *Proceedings of the 9th International Congress on Nutrition,* vol 2. Basel, Switzerland, S Karger AG, 1975, pp 160–167.

2. Beisel WR, Sawyer WD, Ryll ED, et al: Metabolic effects of intracellular infections in man. *Ann Intern Med* 67:744–779, 1967.

3. Moore FD, Oleson KH, McMurrey JD, et al (eds): Acute injury and infection: operation, open trauma, sepsis, burns, fractures, in *The Body Cell Mass and Its Supporting Environment: Body Composition in Health and Disease.* Philadelphia, WB Saunders Company, 1963, pp 224–277.

4. Long CL, Spencer JL, Kinney JM, et al: Carbohydrate metabolism in man: effect of elective operations and major injury. *J Appl Physiol* 31:110–116, 1971.

5. Rayfield EJ, Curnow RT, George DT, et al: Impaired carbohydrate metabolism during a mild viral illness. *N Engl J Med* 298:618–621, 1973.

6. Woolfson *AMJ*, Heatley RV and Allison SP: Insulin to inhibit protein catabolism after injury. *N Engl J Med* 300: 14–17, 1979.

7. Fller JS, Kahn CS and Roth J: Receptors, antirecptor antibodies and oral mechanisms of insulin resistance. *N Engl J Med* 300: 413–419, 1979.

8. Beisel WR, Herman YF, Sauberlich HE, et al: Experimentally induced sandfly fever and vitamin metabolism in man. *Am J Clin Nutr* 25:1165–1173, 1972.

9. Cockerell GL: Changes in plasma protein-bound carbohydrates and glycoprotein patterns during infection, inflammation and starvation. *Proc Soc Exp Biol Med* 142:1072–1076, 1973.

10. Powanda MC, Cockerell GL, Pekarek RS: Amino acid and zinc movement in relation to protein synthesis early in inflammation. *Am J Physiol* 225:399–401, 1973.

11. Rapoport MI, Beisel WR: Studies of tryptophan metabolism in experimental animals and man during infectious illness. *Am J Clin Nutr* 24:807–814, 1971.

12. Beisel WR, Pekarek RS, Wannemacher RW Jr: The impact of infectious disease on trace-element metabolism on the host, in Hoekstra WG, Suttie JW, Ganther HE, et al (eds): *Trace Element Metabolism in Animals,* vol 2. Baltimore, University Park Press, 1974, pp 217–240.

13. Weinberg ED: Iron and susceptibility to infectious disease. *Science* 184:952–956, 1974.

14. Scrimshaw NS, Taylor CE, Gordon JE: *Interactions of Nutrition and Infection,* Monograph No. 57. Geneva, World Health Organization, 1968.

11 Vitamin D in Health and Disease

Hector F. DeLuca, PhD

Calcium is one of the most tightly regulated subtances in the plasma, being held constant at 10 mg/100 ml or 2.5 mM. This remarkable constancy of plasma calcium concentration is of obvious essential importance because of its role in the neuromuscular junction, nerve conduction, muscle contraction, adhesion of one cell to another, membrane permeability, blood clotting, and other functions. Perhaps the most important function is that which occurs at the neuromuscular junction, in which the ambient calcium concentration is critical. In the absence of sufficient amounts of calcium there is a continual excitation at the neuromuscular junction, resulting in the serious state of tetany and convulsions. An important basic concept in calcium homeostasis is that the physiology of the body is so constructed to preserve the plasma calcium concentration at the expense of both the diet and the skeleton.

It is quite impossible to discuss the regulation of plasma calcium concentration without considering the regulation of phosphorus metabolism as well. Less is known about the control of plasma phosphorus concentration than is known about calcium. Nevertheless, they cannot be separated and both will be considered here.

108

There are two basic humoral agents that are involved in the regulation of calcium in the plasma and are responsible for prevention of hypocalcemia. These two agents are vitamin D and parathyroid hormone. Although vitamin D has long been considered as a vitamin, more recent advances have revealed that it is the precursor of at least one hormone involved in the regulation of calcium and phosphorus metabolism. This endocrine system, which is located in the kidney, is perhaps the central one in the regulation of these two ions, assuming a role more important than that of parathyroid hormone. Figure 11-1 illustrates the structure of vitamin D_3 and depicts it as a prohormone. Vitamin D_3 is the natural form of the vitamin formed in the skin upon ultraviolet irradiation. The numbering system is derived from the cholesterol convention and it is important to pay close attention to carbons 25 and 1, which represent the sites of vitamin D activation in its conversion to a hormone. Attention should also be focused on carbon 24, which is the position of another hydroxylation believed at this time to be the primary route for inactivation of the potent vitamin D molecule. Note that the vitamin D compound is a steroid type, although not exactly a steroid since it is missing the B ring.

Figure 11-2 demonstrates the structure of human parathyroid hormone, which has recently been sequenced and its structure completely elucidated. There is some disagreement with regard to two amino acids in the sequence, but not of sufficient importance to be argued here. This hor-

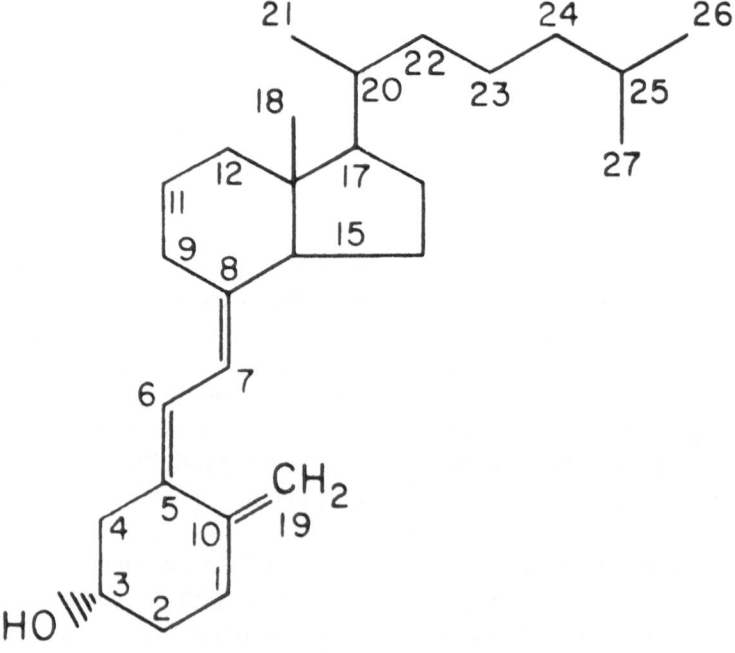

Figure 11-1 Structure of vitamin D_3, the prohormone.

mone is a peptide hormone whose primary functional sequence is in residues 1 - 34. In fact, the 1 - 34 human parathyroid hormone has been chemically synthesized and is available for experimental work; this section of the peptide hormone can carry out all the known functions of the parathyroid hormone. In contrast to the vitamin D system, the parathyroid hormone has an extremely short lifetime and its action is extremely rapid.

In considering the regulation of plasma calcium and phosphorus concentrations, Figure 11-3 provides a diagrammatic sketch. It is first of all important to realize that plasma calcium and phosphorus concentrations are supersaturated with regard to the mineral component of bone. It is also important to realize that the mineral component of bone does not communicate directly with the extracellular fluid compartment. The mineral phase of bone, with its own fluid compartment that bathes the crystals, is separated from the extracellular fluid compartment by a membrane of cells. The bone fluid compartment must be considered to represent the solubility of hydroxyapatite, whereas the extracellular fluid compartment must be considered to represent the plasma levels of calcium and phosphorus. The extracellular fluid compartment therefore has much higher concentrations of both calcium and phosphorus. To maintain these high concentrations, it is necessary to use metabolic energy to pump calcium from the bone fluid compartment to the extracellular fluid compartment, to pump calcium from the intestinal lumen to the extracellular fluid compartment, and finally to pump calcium and phosphorus from the renal tubular fluid to the extracellular fluid compartment.

The cells and their pump systems that pump the calcium and phosphorus into the extracellular fluid compartment are regulated by vitamin D and the parathyroid hormone. Thus it is known that the transport of calcium across the intestine is activated by vitamin D, and indirectly by the parathyroid hormone. The renal transport of calcium is largely independent of both humoral agents, inasmuch as 99% of the filtered calcium is reabsorbed in the absence of either agent. However, the remaining 1% is under the control of vitamin D and the parathyroid hormone working in concert. The pumping of calcium and phosphorus from the bone fluid compartment into the extracellular fluid compartment requires the presence of both vitamin D and parathyroid hormone. It is not known whether the mineralization process is under the control of any agent, although the possible control by some form of vitamin D has been suggested.

We have learned during the past decade that, in order for vitamin D to carry out its role in regulating the calcium and phosphorus pump systems, it must be metabolized to its active forms. Figure 11-4 demonstrates what has been learned about vitamin D metabolism. Normally vitamin D_3 is synthesized in the skin by means of ultraviolet light incident upon the epidermis, which contains 7-dehydrocholesterol. A photolysis reaction occurs in

110

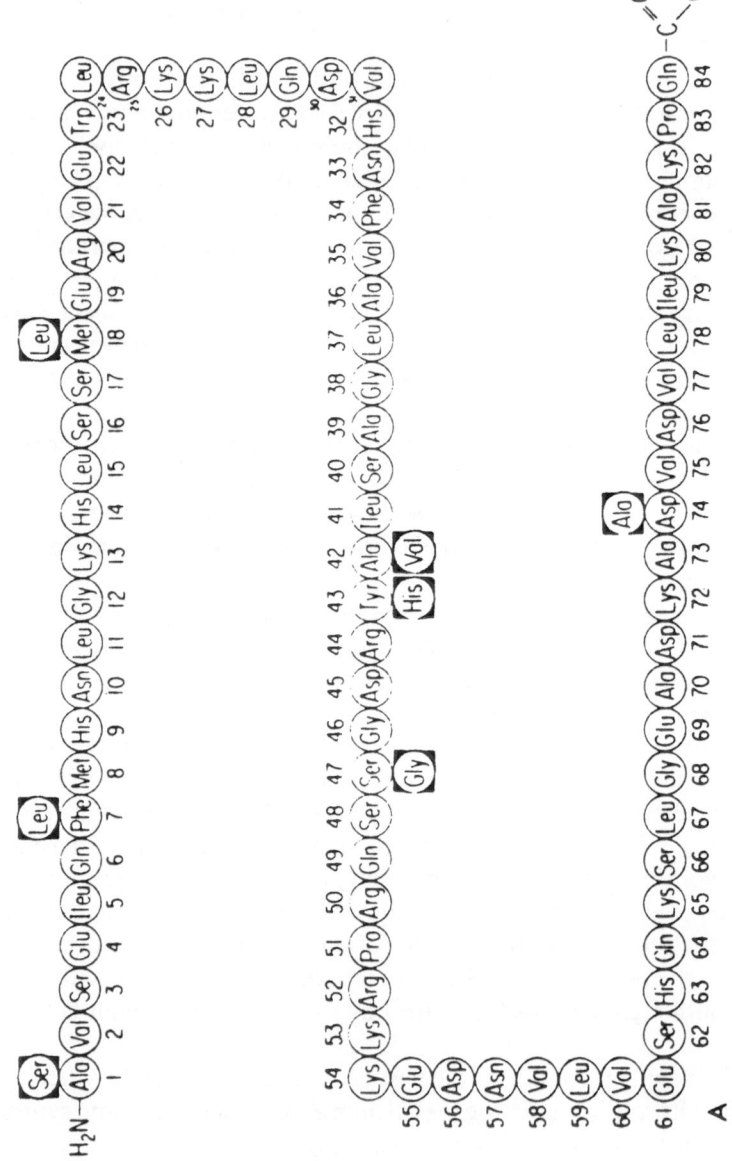

Figure 11-2 Structure of human parathyroid hormone.

which the B ring of 7-dehydrocholesterol is ruptured, yielding vitamin D_3. Vitamin D_3 can also be taken in the diet; it rapidly accumulates in the liver where it undergoes its first obligatory reaction. In the liver it is hydroxylated at carbon 25 to produce the major circulating form of vitamin D, namely 25-hydroxyvitamin D_3(25-OH-D_3). This hydroxylation is somewhat regulated, although the regulation by the product itself can be overcome largely by the administration of larger amounts of vitamin D.

25-Hydroxyvitamin D_3 circulates bound to a 52,000-dalton-α-globulin that is a specific transport protein for the vitamin D molecules. 25-OH-D_3 does not function directly but must be further metabolized at physiologic concentrations. Further metabolism occurs in the kidney, where a specific 25-OH-D_3-1-hydroxylase is found exclusively in renal mitochondria. This hydroxylase inserts a hydroxyl in the 1α position to form $1\alpha,25$-dihydroxyvitamin D_3 ($1\alpha,25$-(OH)$_2$$D_3$). Much is known concerning the enzymology of the 1-hydroxylase and it is this enzyme that is tightly feedback-regulated, as will be demonstrated later. The 1,25-(OH)$_2$$D_3$ is the hormonal form of vitamin D_3 that is transported by the α-globulin to the intestine and bone as well as other sites in the kidney where it carries out its well-known functions. The basic observation, which led to the demonstration that 1,25-(OH)$_2$$D_3$ is the hormonal form of the vitamin and is its active

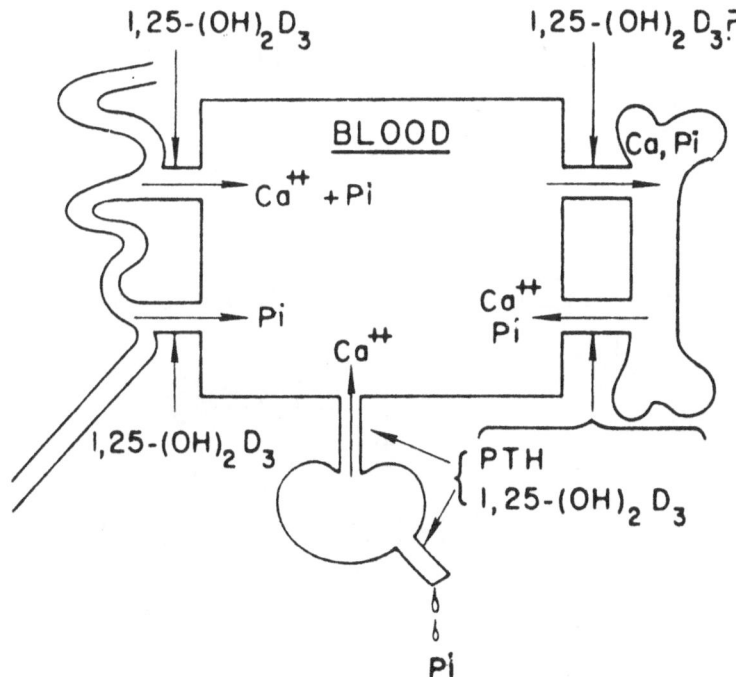

Figure 11-3 Physiologic roles of vitamin D. PTH: parathyroid hormone.

112

form, is shown in Table 11-1. Thus it can be demonstrated that nephrectomy, which prevents the conversion of 25-OH-D₃ to 1,25-(OH)₂D₃, can also prevent the response of intestinal calcium transport, intestinal phosphate transport, and bone calcium mobilization to 25-OH-D₃ and vitamin D₃ but cannot prevent the response to 1,25-(OH)₂D₃. This observation is also of great clinical importance. It demonstrates that the kidney is the exclusive site of synthesis of 1,25-(OH)₂D₃, and furthermore demonstrates that this is an essential reaction for vitamin D function.

In normal animals or normal man there is an alternative to the 1-hydroxylation, namely 24-hydroxylation. This hydroxylation does not occur in vitamin D-deficient animals and it turns out that 1,25-(OH)₂D₃ in-

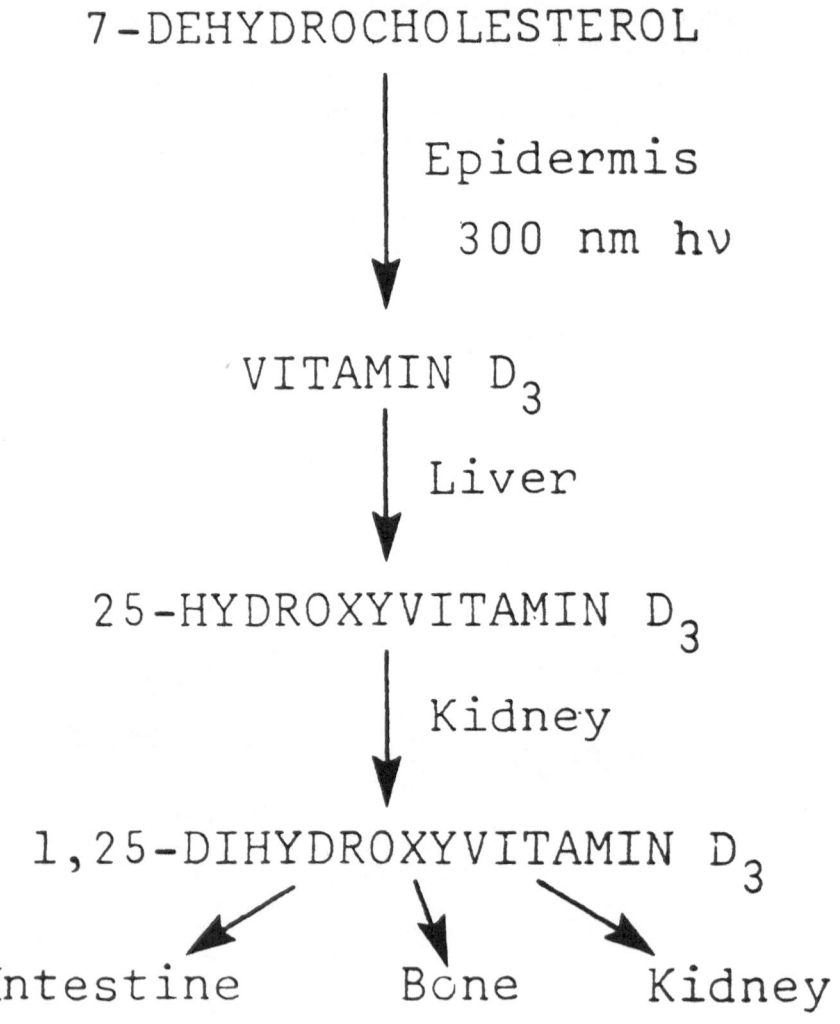

Figure 11-4 Intermediates in the metabolism of vitamin D.

Table 11-1
The Role of the Kidney in 1,25-(OH)₂D₃ Synthesis

	1,25-(OH)$_2$D$_3$ Synthesis	Stimulation of Calcium 25-OH-D$_3$	Absorption by 1,25-(OH)$_2$D$_3$
No renal tissue	--	--	+ + +
Acutely impaired renal function	+ + +	+ +	+ + +

duces the appearance of this hydroxylase, which inserts an hydroxyl on carbon 24 of either 25-OH-D$_3$ or 1,25-(OH)$_2$D$_3$. The exact function of the 24-hydroxylation remains in doubt, although current evidence suggests that it is the first signal for inactivation of the vitamin D molecule. Certainly the 24-hydroxylated vitamins in the chick are much less active than their non–24-hydroxylated vitamins, as shown in Figure 11-5. Thus normal animals and humans have available to them the alternate of either 1-hydroxylating 25-OH-D$_3$ or 24-hydroxylating 25-OH-D$_3$.

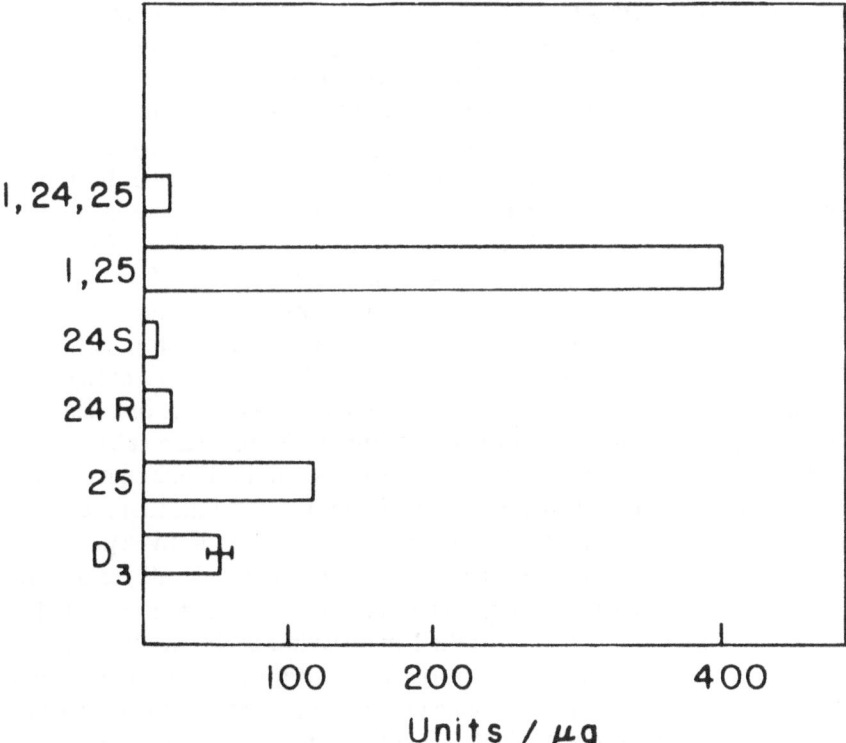

Figure 11-5 The biologic activity of D$_3$ metabolites in chicks. The R and S refer to stereochemical configuration of the 24-hydroxyl group.

As shown in figure 11-6, conversion of 25-OH-D$_3$ to 1,25-(OH)$_2$D$_3$ is under control of serum calcium concentration either directly or indirectly. At normal serum calcium concentrations both 24,25-(OH)$_2$D$_3$ and 1,25-(OH)$_2$D$_3$ are made. However, under conditions of even slight hypocalcemia there is a stimulation of the 25-OH-D$_3$-1-hydroxylase and the appearance of its product in the plasma, and a shut down of the 24-hydroxylation. Conversely, under conditions of hypercalcemia the calcium-mobilizing hormone, 1,25-(OH)$_2$D$_3$, is not made and instead, 24-hydroxylation of the vitamin D molecules occurs. This plot clearly demonstrates the hormonal nature of 1,25-(OH)$_2$D$_3$, the major calcium-mobilizing hormone.

It is the parathyroid gland that is the calcium-sensing organ of the body, as shown in Figure 11-7. Under conditions of hypocalcemia the parathyroid glands secrete the peptide hormone, parathyroid hormone, and it has been demonstrated in our group that the parathyroid hormone stimulates production of 1,25-(OH)$_2$D$_3$ by some unknown mechanism. The 1,25-(OH)$_2$D$_3$ then proceeds to the intestine, kidney, and bone where it initiates calcium transport mechanisms. In the intestine, parathyroid hormone does not function directly but rather functions by stimulating production of 1,25-(OH)$_2$D$_3$. At the bone site both 1,25-(OH)$_2$D$_3$ and the parathyroid hormone are required at physiologic concentrations for mobilizing calcium. This is also likely to be the case for renal tubular reabsorption of calcium. Figure 11-8 demonstrates the calcium homeostatic mechanism as it is now understood. In response to even slight hypocalcemia the parathyroid glands secrete the 84-amino-acid peptide hormone, parathyroid hormone, which is transported rapidly to the kidney and bone. It does not bind to small intestine. In the kidney, besides causing a phosphate diuresis and improving renal reabsorption of calcium, it stimulates production of 1,25-(OH)$_2$D$_3$. This compound proceeds to the intestine where it stimulates the transport of calcium across intestinal epithelium. At the bone site, both 1,25-(OH)$_2$D$_3$ and the parathyroid hormone are required. These mechanisms cause the appearance of calcium in the extracellular fluid compartment, causing a rise in serum calcium concentration, which in turn shuts off the parathyroid hormone signal.

There are two mechanisms of calcium homeostasis; the first is a short-term mechanism and the other is a longer-term mechanism. In response to a single perturbation in serum calcium concentration the parathyroid gland secretes the parathyroid hormone very rapidly, which is rapidly bound to kidney and bone. The response of the 1-hydroxylase to the parathyroid hormone is very slow; instead, on a short-term basis the parathyroid hormone stimulates renal reabsorption of calcium and mobilization of bone calcium with existing 1,25-(OH)$_2$D$_3$. This provides a short-term correction of the hypocalcemia, but if there is chronic hypocalcemia there is continual stimulation of the kidney, which responds by secreting 1,25-(OH)$_2$D$_3$ over a

115

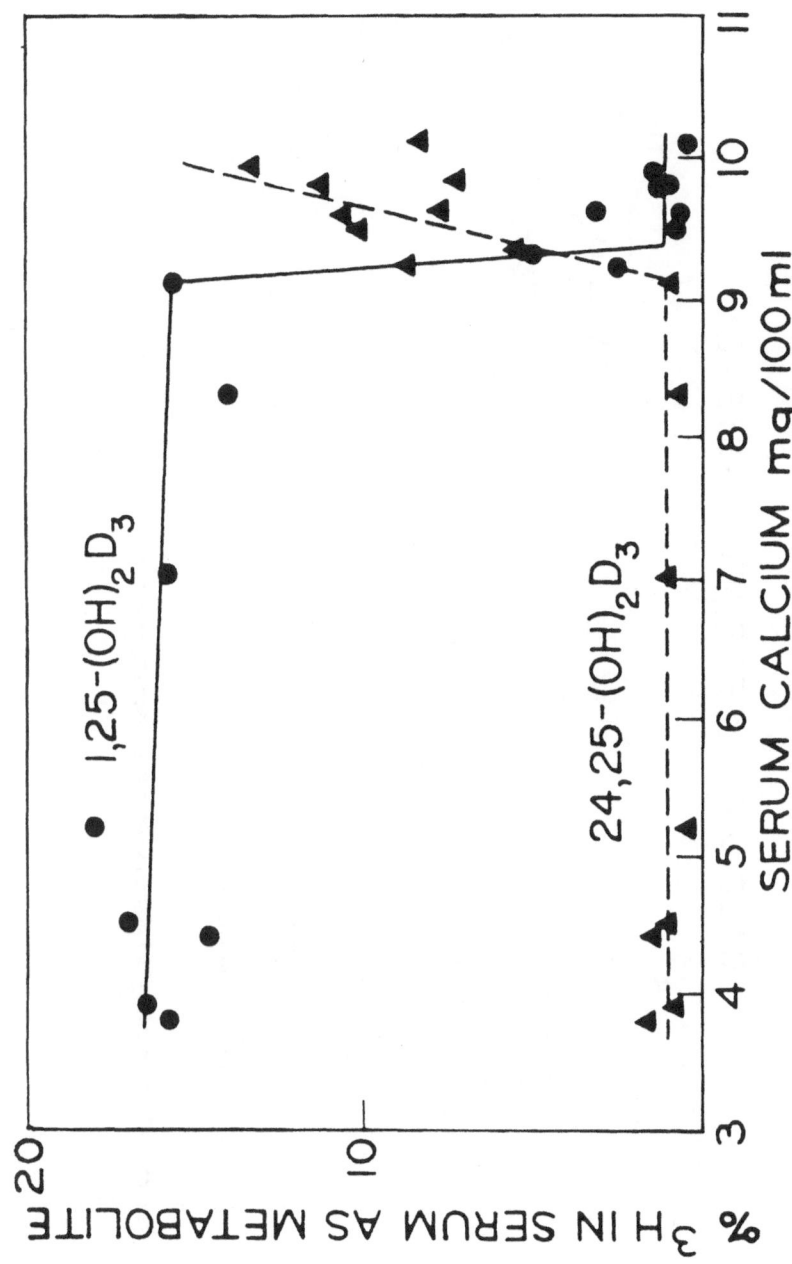

Figure 11-6 The effect of serum calcium concentrations on the conversion of 25-OH-D₃ to 1,25-(OH)₂D₃.

116

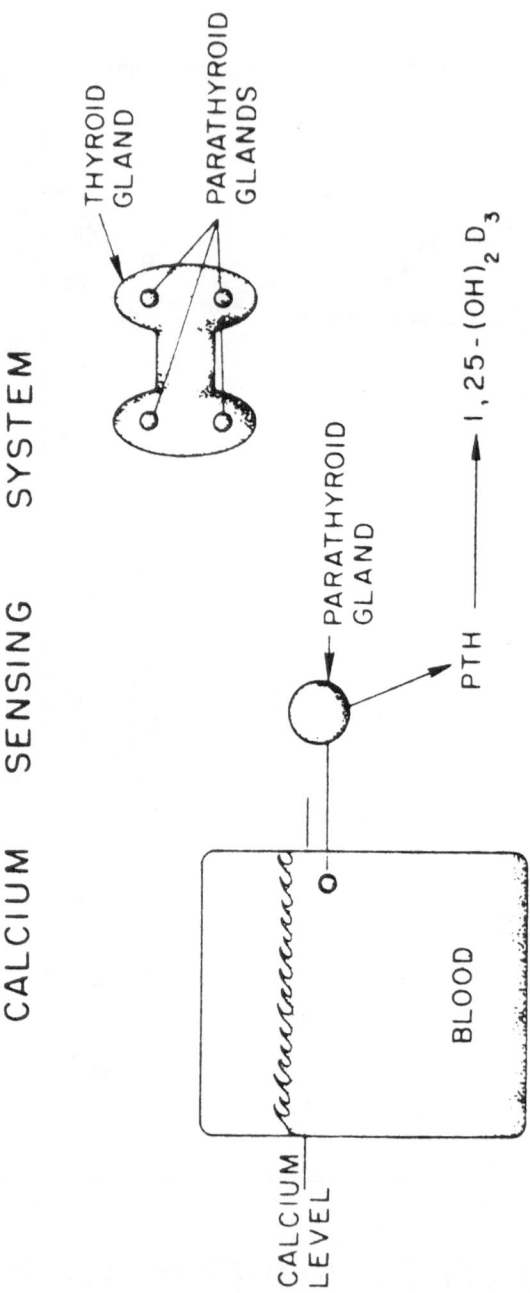

Figure 11-7 The parathyroid gland as the calcium-sensing organ of the body. PTH: parathyroid hormone.

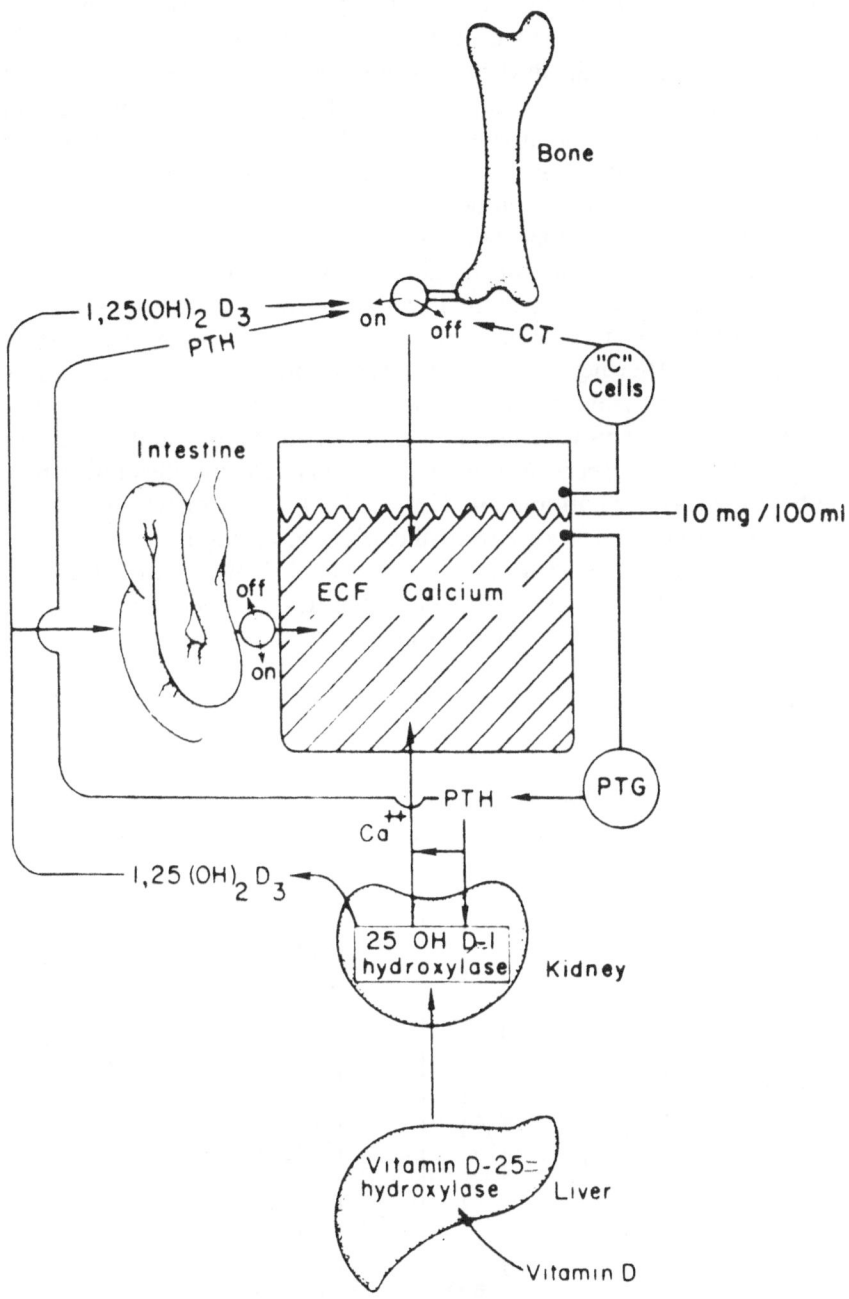

Figure 11-8 Schematic representation of the homeostatic mechanism regulating calcium metabolism. PTH: parathyroid hormone; CT: calcitonin; "C" cells: calcitonin-secreting cells; ECF: extracellular fluid; PTG: parathyroid glands.

period of hours. The 1,25-(OH)$_2$D$_3$ then appears in intestine, bone, and kidney. In the bone and kidney it increases the sensitivity to parathyroid hormone, whereas in the intestine it stimulates the intestine by itself to a high efficiency of calcium absorption, providing an important mechanism for the body to sequester needed calcium from the environment. In the absence of the ability to increase intestinal calcium absorption to meet the body's needs, the skeleton will be sacrificed, which probably provides an important factor in the appearance of osteoporosis.

The ability of the intestine to adapt to low- and high-calcium diets is shown in Figure 11-9; furthermore, it can be shown when an exogenous and saturating amount of 1,25-(OH)$_2$D$_3$ is supplied, the ability of the intestine to adapt its efficiency of calcium absorption to dietary calcium is eliminated. Parathyroidectomized animals given a constant exogenous supply of parathyroid hormone also show a lack of ability to modulate their intestinal calcium transport in response to dietary calcium, illustrating that both the parathyroid hormone and 1,25-(OH)$_2$D$_3$ are intimately involved in the signal for adjustment of intestinal calcium absorption.

Another important calcium need is signaled during the period of reproduction, which is especially evident in birds whose eggs are laid with a heavily calcified shell. The requirement for calcium during this process is

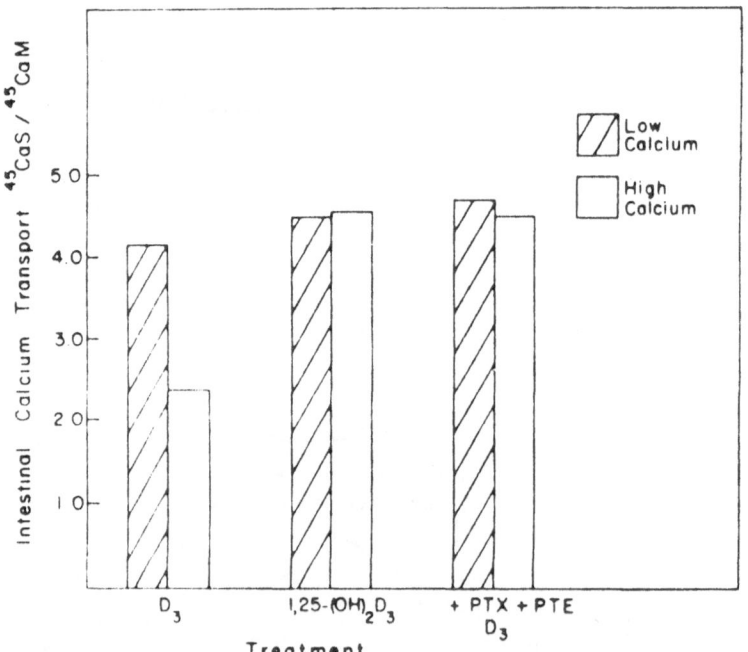

Figure 11-9 Elimination of intestinal calcium adaptation by 1,25-(OH)$_2$D$_3$ or parathyroid hormone. PTX: parathyroidectomy; PTE: parathyroid extract; CaS:^{45}Ca on serosal surface; CaM: ^{45}Ca on mucosal surface.

immense, and has led us to examine the question of what initiates the formation of medullary bone and the resorption of medullary bone during eggshell formation. This has led to the demonstration that estradiol has a marked stimulatory effect on the 25-OH-D_3-1-hydroxylase in birds. This stimulation requires the presence of testosterone and/or progesterone. In adult male birds having adequate levels of testosterone injected with estradiol there is a marked enhancement of the 25-OH-D_3-1-hydroxylase and a shutdown of the 24-hydroxylase, as shown in Figure 11-10; this is followed by a rise in plasma calcium concentration to very high levels. Similar control by estradiol of the 1-hydroxylase in mammals may also be true. Thus the sex hormones provide an important regulator of the 25-OH-D_3-1-hydroxylase.

It is now important to apply this understanding of the hydroxylases to certain disease states of interest to orthopedic surgeons. The first and most critical is that of the hypoparathyroid patients (Figure 11-11). These patients are very nicely managed by an exogenous source of 1,25-$(OH)_2D_3$ or its analog 1α-hydroxyvitamin D_3 (1α-OH-D_3), plus sufficient amounts of oral calcium to use the intestine as the primary mechanism for adjusting calcium in the serum. Pseudohypoparathyroids, who differ because their target organs are resistant to their own parathyroid hormone which is secreted normally or in excess by these patients, are managed in a similar way.

An important and widespread disease is osteoporosis, which is poorly understood, is probably a heterogeneous disease, and undoubtedly has a very diverse origin. Figure 11-12 illustrates the factors that are known to be involved; note that a failure to absorb sufficient amounts of calcium to meet the body's needs will result in sacrifice of the skeleton. The demonstration that circulating levels of 1,25-$(OH)_2D_3$ diminish with age and have a tendency to be lower in diagnosed osteoporotics, suggests that an inability to make sufficient amounts of 1,25-$(OH)_2D_3$ may contribute to the failure of intestinal calcium absorption over the course of many years. This would lead to a reliance on the skeleton for calcium to support serum calcium concentration. Thus the skeleton is sacrificed, giving rise to osteoporosis. It is therefore possible that the administration of the 1-hydroxylated vitamins will help prevent the development of the disease, although it is possible that its administration can help in the treatment of already diseased patients.

As described above, 1,25-$(OH)_2D_3$ plays an important role in stimulating the transport of phosphate, at least in the small intestine and perhaps elsewhere, since the rise in serum phosphorus is the primary mechanism involved in the healing of rachitic lesions in rats and in children. An important function of 1,25-$(OH)_2D_3$, therefore, is to elevate plasma phosphorus concentration. Figure 11-13 shows that plasma phosphorus concentration even in thyroparathyroidectomized animals exerts a marked control on the accumulation of 1,25-$(OH)_2D_3$ in the plasma. Thus, as

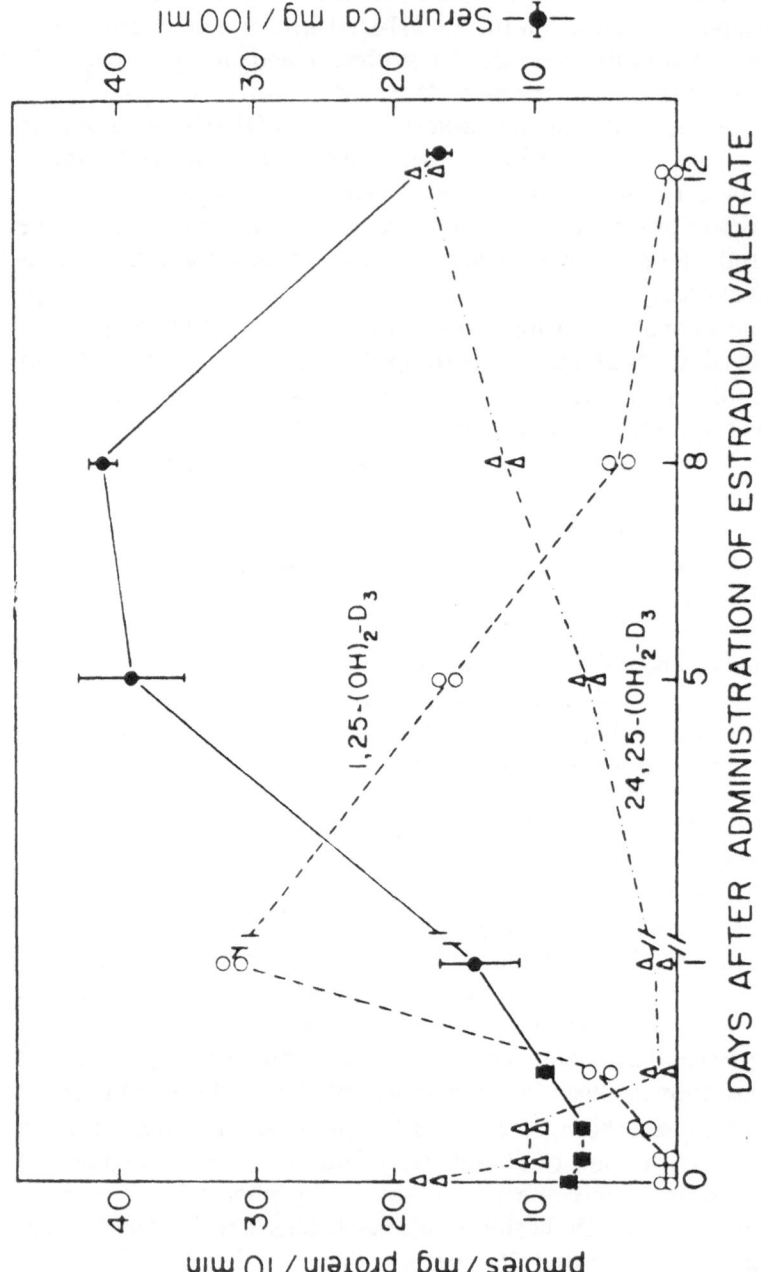

Figure 11-10 The effect of estradiol valerate administration on serum calcium, 1,25-(OH)₂D₃, and 24,25-(OH)₂D₃ levels.

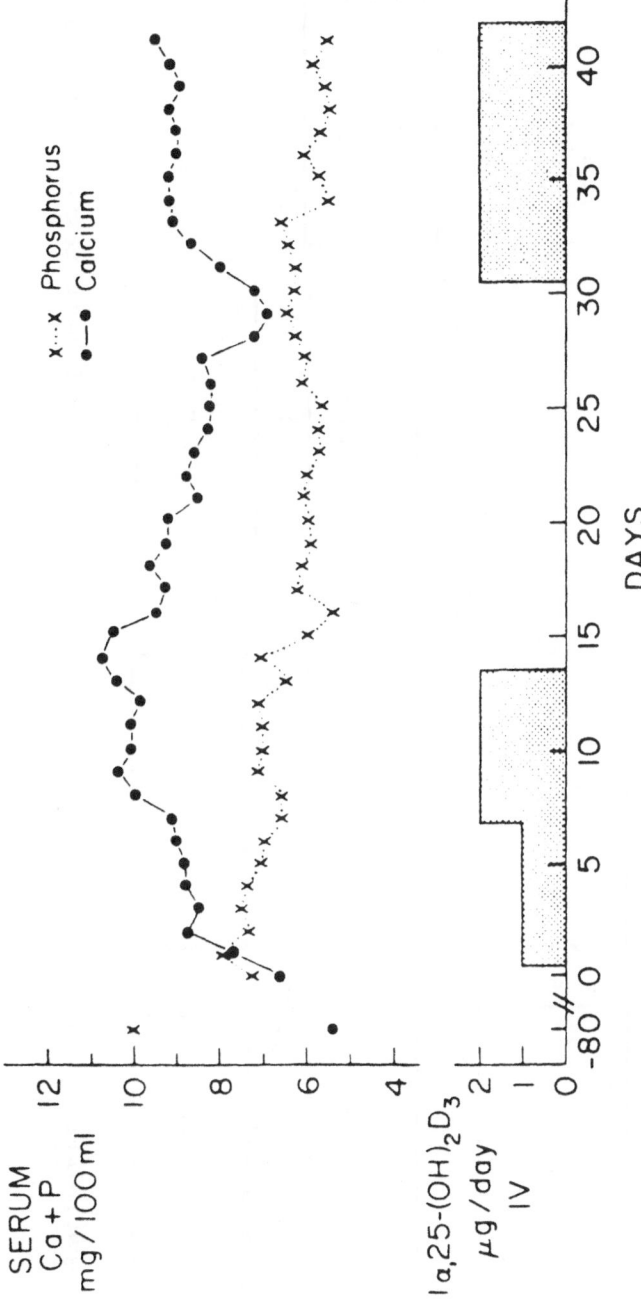

Figure 11-11 The effect of $1\alpha,25\text{-}(OH)_2D_3$ administration on serum phosphorus and calcium levels in hypoparathyroid patients.

122

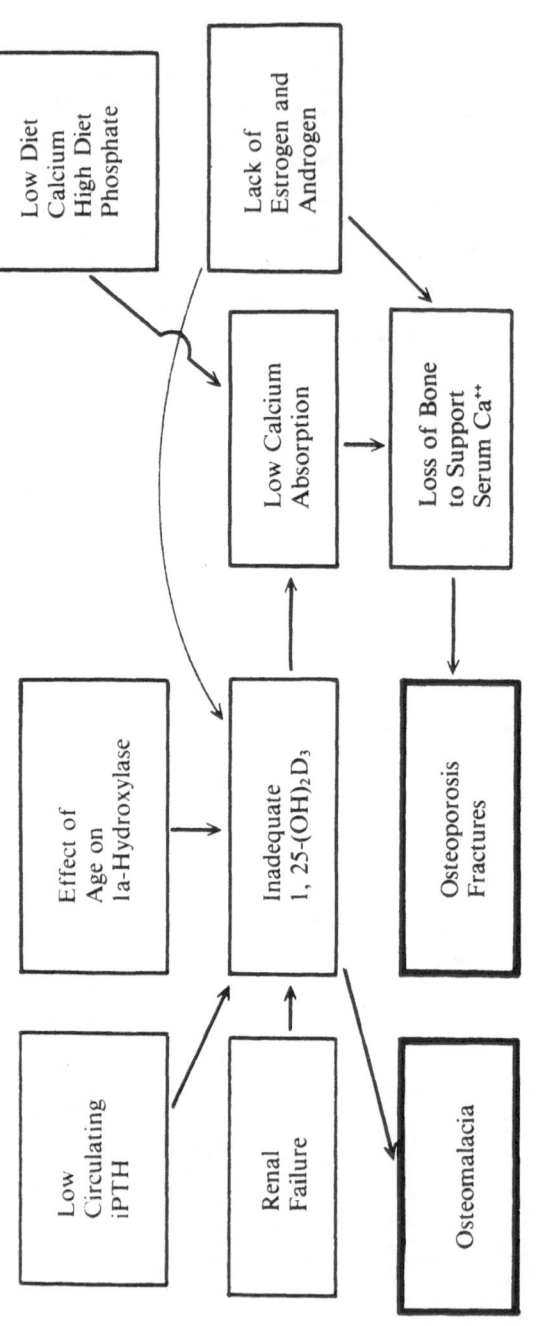

Figure 11-12 Factors involved in the pathogenesis of osteoporosis and osteomalacia. iPTH: immunoreactive parathyroid hormone.

hypophosphatemia is induced by phosphate deprivation, there is a stimulation of $1,25\text{-}(OH)_2D_3$ in the plasma. This is the result of increased 25-OH-D_3-1-hydroxylase and other factors. $1,25\text{-}(OH)_2D_3$, therefore, can be considered as a phosphate-controlling hormone as well as a calcium-controlling hormone.

Figure 11-14 demonstrates a hypothesis that has been suggested to invoke known mechanisms in the regulation of the 25-OH-D_3-1-hydroxylase; namely, phosphate depletion on the one hand and parathyroid hormone on the other. Both lead to a diminution of the renal cell level of inorganic phosphorus: the parathyroid hormone by blocking phosphate reabsorption, and phosphate deprivation by providing less phosphate to be reabsorbed. It is therefore possible that the renal cell level of inorganic phosphate is the underlying mechanism controlling the 1-hydroxylase. This is a hypothesis that will require further verification.

Figure 11-15 illustrates the mechanisms involved in renal osteodystrophy, in which there is a failure to produce $1,25\text{-}(OH)_2D_3$ either by lack of renal mass or by high ambient phosphate concentrations. This leads to an impaired intestinal absorption of calcium and eventually to a resistance of the bone to secreted parathyroid hormone, giving rise to secondary hyperparathyroidism, osteomalacia, and severe bone disease. It is now well-known that administration of $1,25\text{-}(OH)_2D_3$, at least in most cases, will reverse the lesions of bone, provided the serum phosphorus concentration is first adjusted to normal and provided the patient does not have autonomous parathyroid glands.

Finally, some comments should be made about vitamin D-resistant rickets. One group of patients is believed to have a specific block in the gene that expresses the renal 25-OH-D_3-1-hydroxylase; this is the autosomal recessive vitamin D-dependency syndrome described by Prader and by Fraser.[1,2] Figure 11-16 illustrates the plasma levels of $1,25\text{-}(OH)_2D_3$ in this disease, which can be managed easily by large doses of vitamin D. The management by large doses of vitamin D is not the result of increased biogenesis of $1,25\text{-}(OH)_2D_3$, but rather the large circulating levels of 25-OH-D_3, which acts as an analog of $1,25\text{-}(OH)_2D_3$. In any case, $1,25\text{-}(OH)_2D_3$ at physiologic concentrations will cure this disease.

The major vitamin D-resistant rachitic condition is the X-linked dominant familial hypophosphatemia, which has been characterized as having a phosphate leak which is resistant to vitamin D and $1,25\text{-}(OH)_2D_3$. This disease is probably a defect in phosphate transport mechanisms; recently we have been privileged to receive mice having this disease from the Bar Harbor Laboratories, and their intestinal phosphate transport mechanism shows a clear resistance to $1,25\text{-}(OH)_2D_3$ (Figure 11-17). Note in normal mice the time course of response of phosphate transport to $1,25\text{-}(OH)_2D_3$ is very long, requiring 18 hours. We have recently discovered a further metabolic system that converts $1,25\text{-}(OH)_2D_3$ to an unknown

124

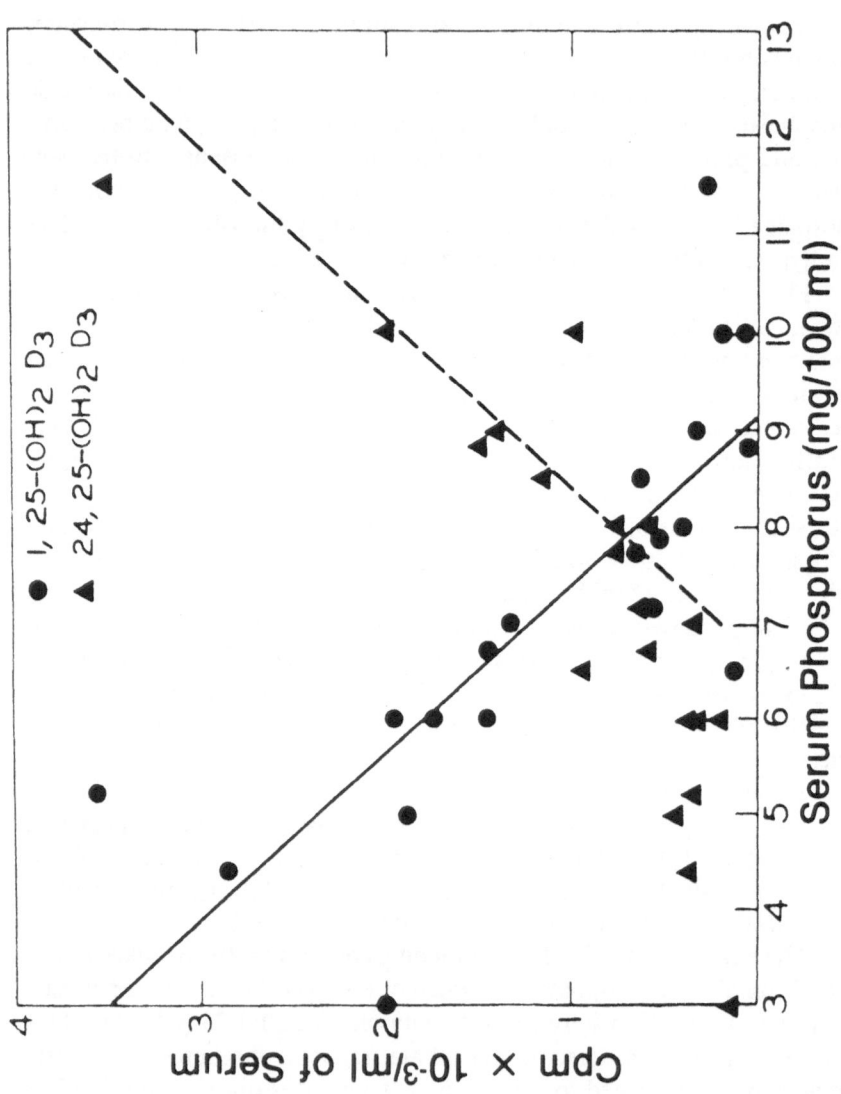

Figure 11-13 The effect of plasma phosphorus levels on plasma 1,25-(OH)₂D₃ in thyroparathyroidectomized animals.

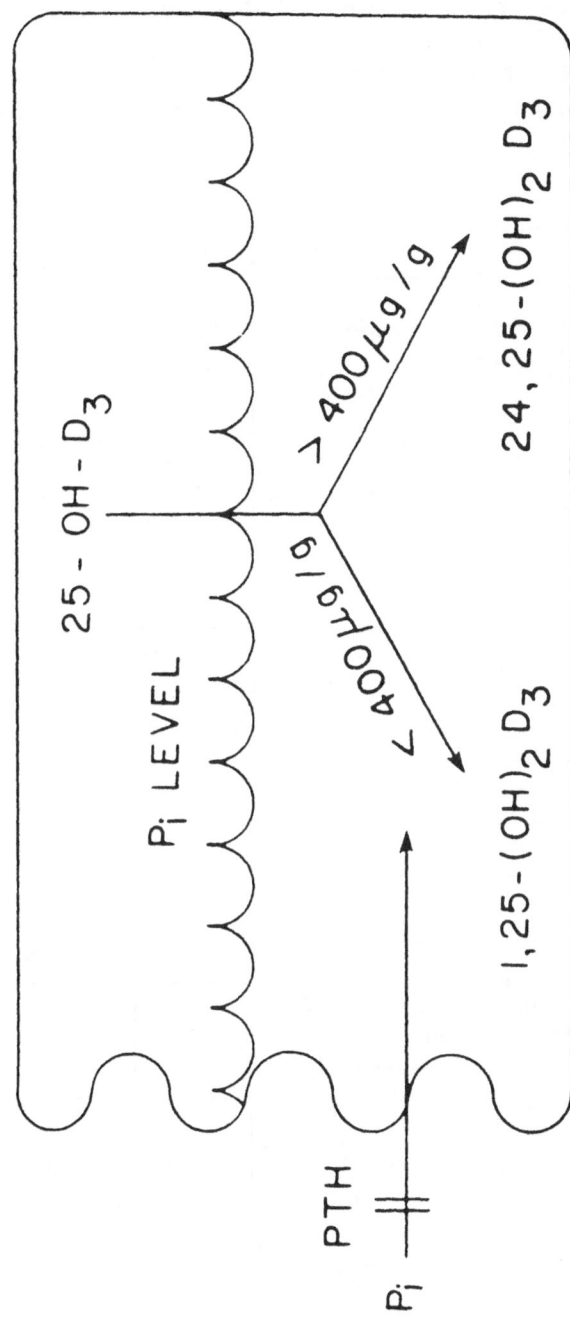

Figure 11-14 Regulation of 1,25-(OH)₂D₃ synthesis in renal cells by inorganic phosphorus. PTH: parathyroid hormone.

126

metabolite(s), with its terminal side chain being oxidized to carbon dioxide and water (Figure 11-18). This illustrates the point that the vitamin D story is not yet completed, and it is very possible that additional hormonal forms of the vitamin will be described.

It is clear that the vitamin D metabolic systems have provided an important new insight into the regulation of calcium and phosphorus metabolism and, most important, have provided new agents that can be

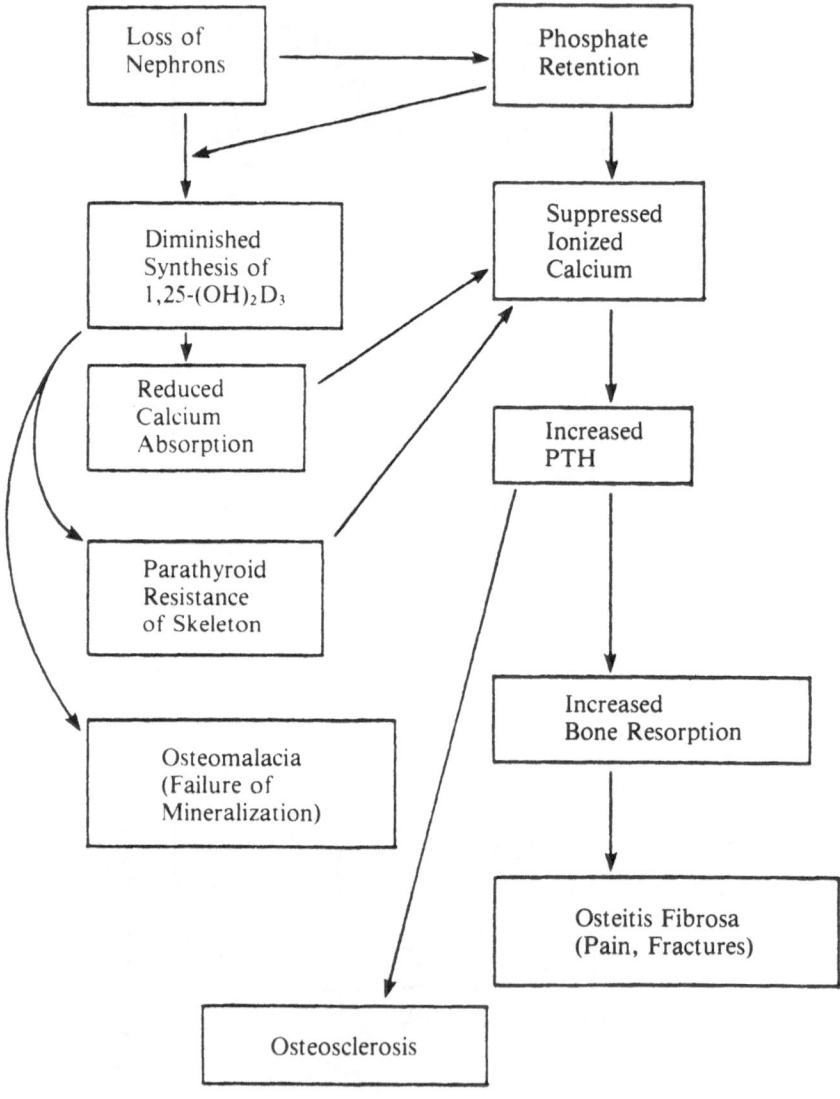

Figure 11-15 Mechanisms involved in renal osteodystrophy. PTH: parathyroid hormone.

used in the treatment of metabolic bone diseases such as renal osteodystrophy, hypoparathyroidism, vitamin D-resistant rickets, and perhaps some types of osteoporosis.

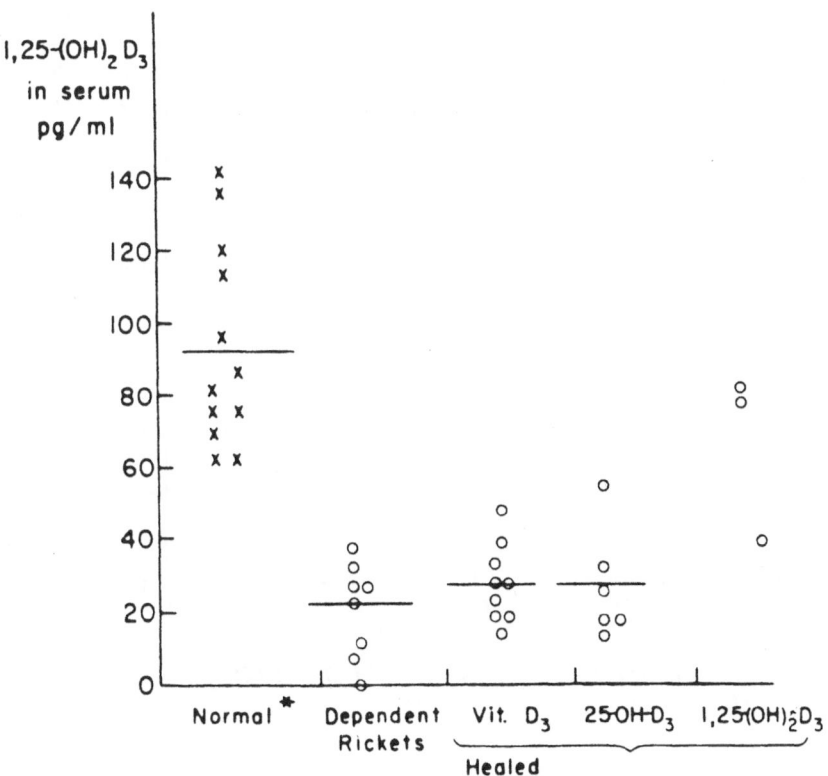

Figure 11-16 The effect of large doses of vitamin D on plasma 1,25-(OH)$_2$D$_3$ in vitamin D dependency syndromes. *Under 12 years of age.

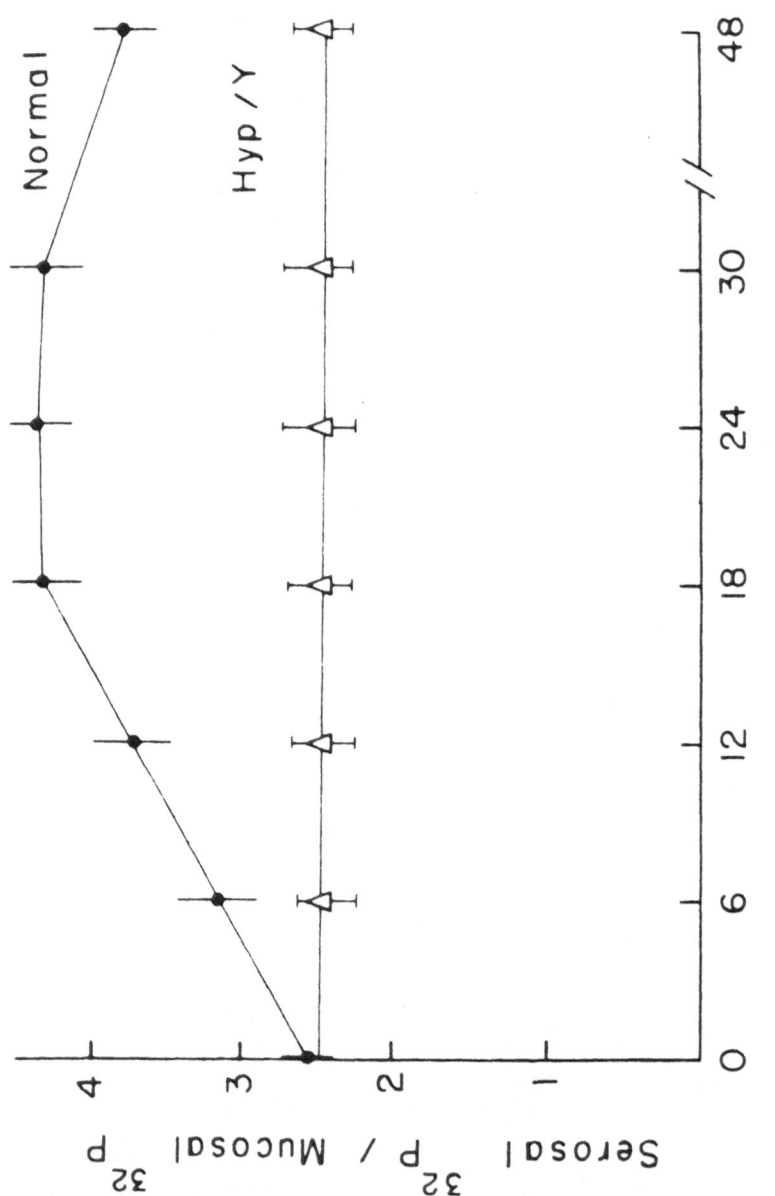

Figure 11-17 The lack of effect of 1,25-(OH)$_2$D$_3$ on phosphate transport in the vitamin D-resistant rachitic condition of the X-linked dominant familial hypophospatemia (Hyp/Y) in mice.

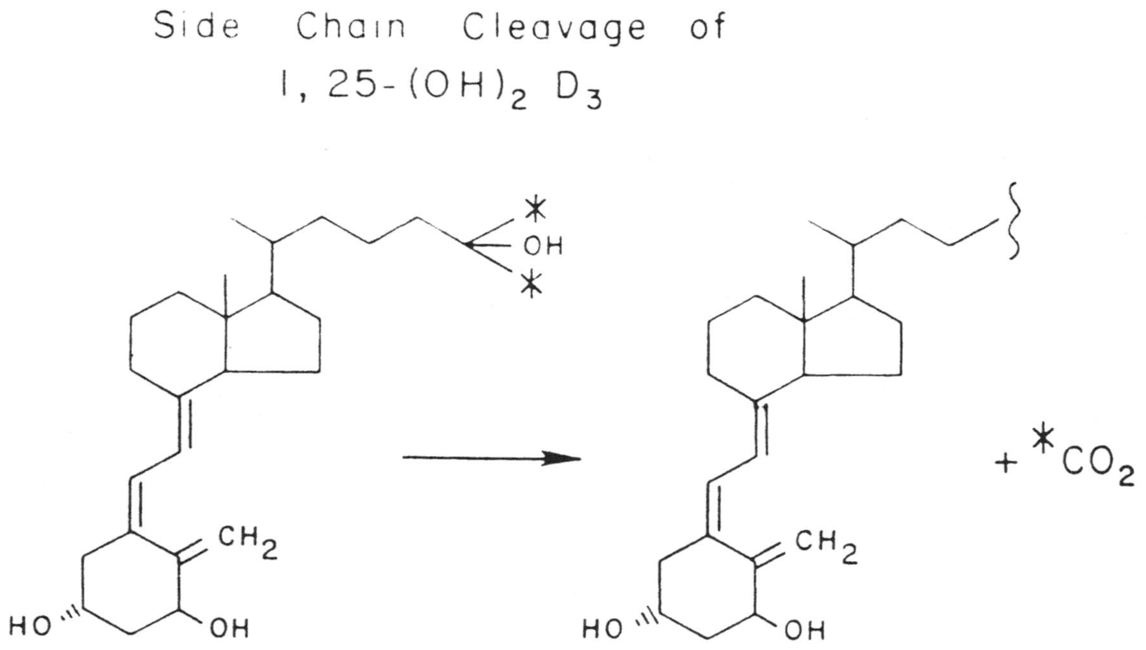

Side Chain Cleavage of
1,25-(OH)$_2$ D$_3$

Figure 11-18 A further metabolite of 1,25-(OH)$_2$D$_3$ — is this a new functional metabolite or a degradation product?

REFERENCES

1. Prader A, Illig R, Heierli E: Eine besondere Form der primaren Vitamin D-resistenten Rachitis mit Hypocalcamie und Autosonal-dominantem Erbang; die hereditare Pseudomangelrachitis. *Helv Paediatr Acta* 16:452–468, 1961.

2. Fraser D, Kooh SW, Kind HP, et al: Pathogenesis of hereditary vitamin D-dependent rickets: an inborn error of vitamin D metabolism involving defective conversion or 25-hydroxyvitamin D to 1,25-dihydroxyvitamin D. *N Engl J Med* 289:817, 1973.

12   Prothrombin Biosynthesis – A Vitamin K-Dependent Reaction

John W. Suttie, PhD

The association between vitamin K and hemostasis was first recognized by Dam in the late 1920s when he characterized 2-methyl-3-phytyl-1,4-naphthoquinone or vitamin K_1, as an antihemorrhagic factor for chicks. The structures of vitamin K_1 and other compounds relevant to this discussion are shown in Figure 12-1. It was originally thought that the only defect in vitamin K deficiency was a lack of plasma prothrombin. During the 1950s it was recognized that there are a large number of plasma factors in addition to prothrombin associated with thrombin generation; subsequently factors X, IX, and VII were identified and shown to be vitamin K-dependent. A diagrammatic representation of the cascade model for blood coagulation as it is currently understood is shown in Figure 12-2. In this scheme, a series of proteins acts as substrates for proteases that convert them to active proteolytic enzymes, which then become the proteases of the next stage of the cascade. Knowledge of the cellular events responsible for the production of prothrombin, the role of vitamin K in this process, and its antagonism by coumarins has come largely from investigations spanning the last ten years. These studies have shown that prothrombin is formed in the liver by a vitamin K-dependent

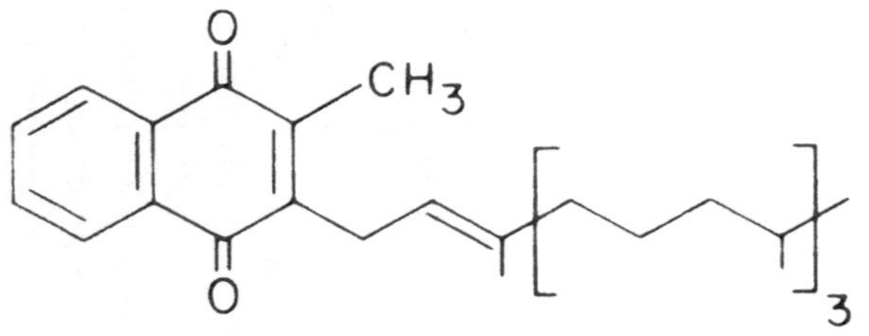

Vitamin K_1

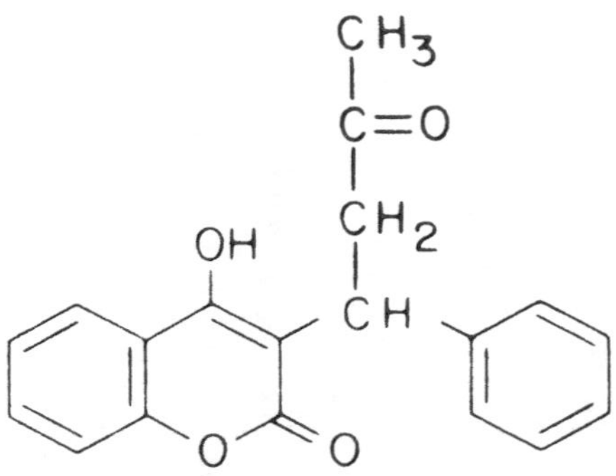

Warfarin

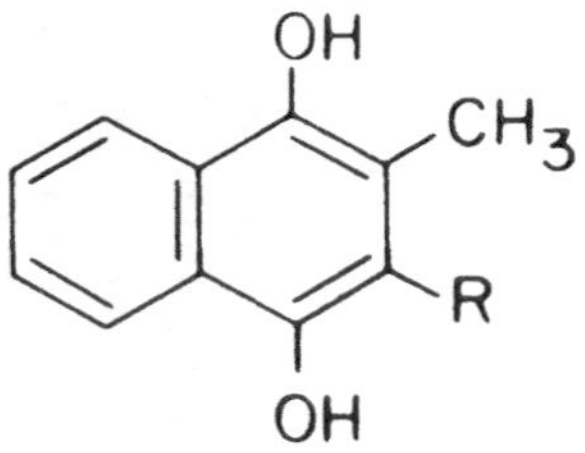

Reduced Vitamin K
(KH_2)

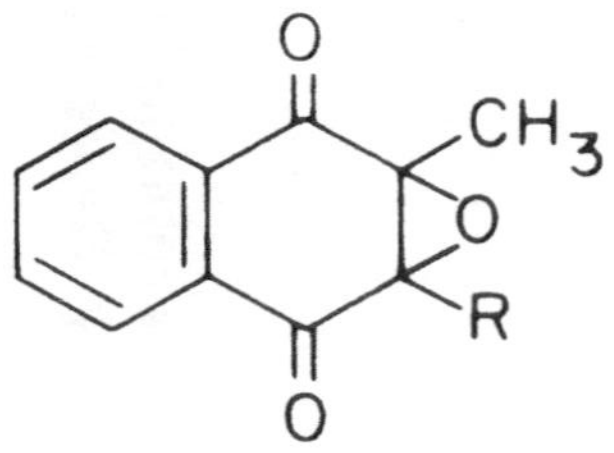

Vitamin K-2,3-epoxide
(Vitamin K oxide)

Figure 12-1 The structures of vitamin K_1 and related compounds.

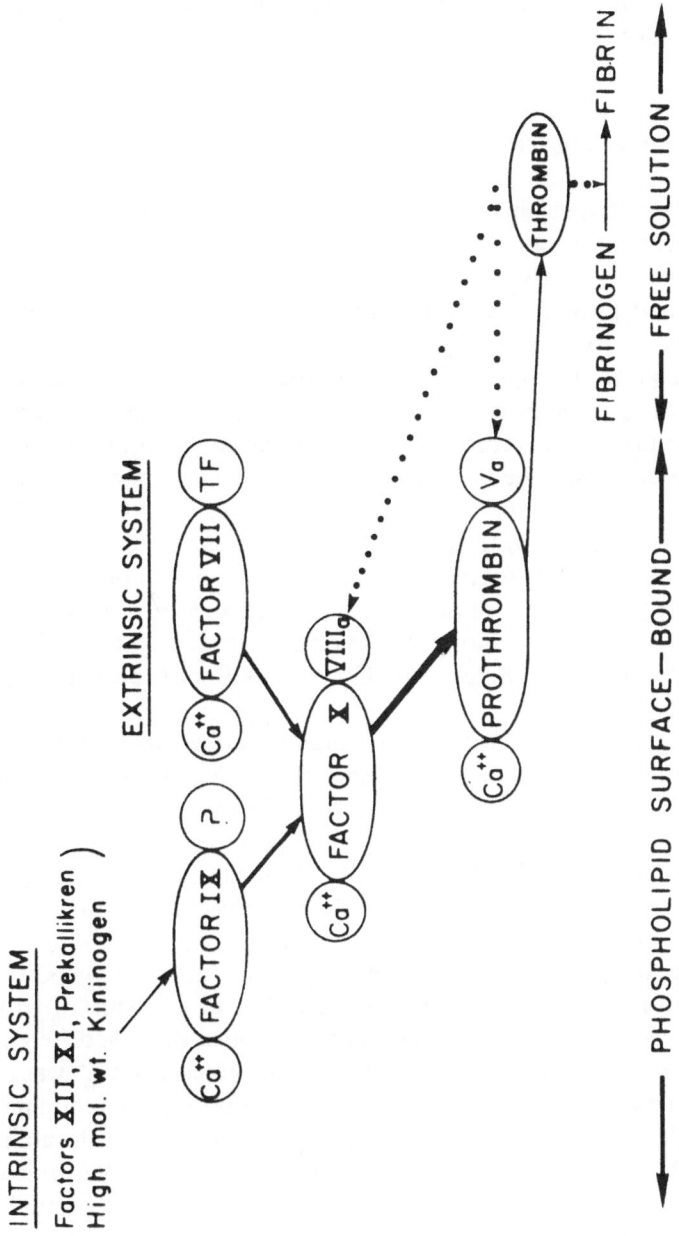

Figure 12-2 A diagrammatic representation of the cascade model for blood coagulation. TF: thrombin formation.

carboxylation of a liver precursor protein. This process and detailed information on the chemistry and activation of prothrombin have recently been reviewed,[1] and only a limited number of specific references will be provided here.

Prothrombin Characterization

The realization that prothrombin was synthesized by a vitamin K-dependent conversion of an inactive liver precursor to active prothrombin came about through biochemical studies of vitamin K-deficient animals[2] and through the investigation of an antigenically similar, but biologically inactive, form of plasma prothrombin found in patients receiving anticoagulant therapy.[3,4] This "abnormal" prothrombin could also be found in the plasma of cattle fed coumarin anticoagulants,[5] and a comparative study of this protein, and of normal bovine prothrombin, was utilized to determine the metabolic role of vitamin K. It was shown that normal prothrombin, but not the abnormal form, has an electrophoretic mobility that is altered by the presence of Ca^{++} ions in the buffer. Following this observation, it was found that normal prothrombin bound Ca^{++} did so cooperatively, ie, in a fashion indicating that special protein structure changes were occurring during the binding process, where the abnormal prothrombin bound relatively little Ca^{++} and did not show evidence of a special cooperative process.

A series of investigations by Suttie and Nelsestuen, and Stenflo and his collaborators (see reference 1) established that the two forms of prothrombin were indistinguishable in molecular weight, amino acid composition after acid hydrolysis, and carbohydrate composition. Although the abnormal prothrombin was essentially inactive in the normal two-stage assay, it could be activated to thrombin by specific snake venom enzymes. Furthermore, the thrombin formed from either form of prothrombin was indistinguishable in biologic activity, indicating that the thrombin portion of the prothrombin molecule was not defective as a result of vitamin K-antagonist effects in cattle. Stenflo demonstrated that the difference in electrophoretic mobility of prothrombins in the presence of Ca^{++} was a property of a fragment of the prothrombin molecule at the amino-terminal end of the molecule. At about the same time, it was shown[6] that the ability of prothrombin to bind to phospholipid was due to a property of this same fragment, now called prothrombin fragment 1. Nelsestuen and Suttie isolated a Ca^{++}-binding peptide from tryspin-digested normal prothrombin that could not be isolated from the abnormal prothrombin molecule; this further limited the vitamin K-dependent modification to a smaller portion of the prothrombin structure. The specific structural difference between normal and abnormal prothrombins was shown by Stenflo and his collaborators[7] and independently by Nelsestuen et al[8] to be the presence of additional carboxyl groups on some of the glutamic acid residues in a peptide from the fragment 1 region of the prothrombin molecule. The structure of this new amino acid, formed as a result of the addition of the extra carboxyl group, γ-carboxyglutamic acid, and its location in the prothrombin molecule are shown in Figure 12-3.

Isolation of Liver Prothrombin-Precursor Proteins

Studies of the abnormal bovine plasma prothrombin suggested that the hypothesized liver precursor might have similar properties and that it should be possible to isolate it. Two proteins have now been isolated[9,10] from the liver of warfarin-treated rats that have the properties predicted for this precursor. The first (precursor I) is a glycoprotein immunochemically similar to prothrombin with a molecular weight indistinguishable from rat prothrombin, which is less negatively charged (pI = 5.8) than prothrombin (pI = 5.0). Specific proteolysis of precursor I yields fragments indistinguishable from those formed by similar proteolysis of prothrombin. This protein does not absorb to $BaSO_4$, its rate of activation by factor X_a and Ca^{++} is not stimulated by phospholipid, and it appears to be identical to prothrombin with the exception that it does not contain sialic acid residues and does not contain γ-carboxyglutamic acid. A second protein with properties very similar, but with an isoelectric point of 7.2, has been isolated from the same microsomal preparations. The increased basic nature of this protein is a property of the amino-terminal region of the molecule, but the chemical alteration responsible for the shift in pH has not yet been determined. The properties of these proteins are summarized in Table 12-1.

Table 12-1
Properties of Rat Plasma Prothrombin and Rat Liver Precursor

Property	Prothrombin	Precursor I	Precursor II
Molecular weight (SDS gel)	85,000	85,000	85,000
pI	5.0	5.8	7.2
Neutral sugars	Yes	Yes	Yes
Sialic acid	Yes	No	No
Phospholipid	Yes	No	No
Adsorbs to $BaSO_4$	Yes	No	No
Thrombin generation (Ca^{++}, PL, X_aV)*	Yes	No	No
Thrombin generation (snake venoms)	Yes	Yes	Yes

*PL: Phospholipid; X_a: factor X_a.

136

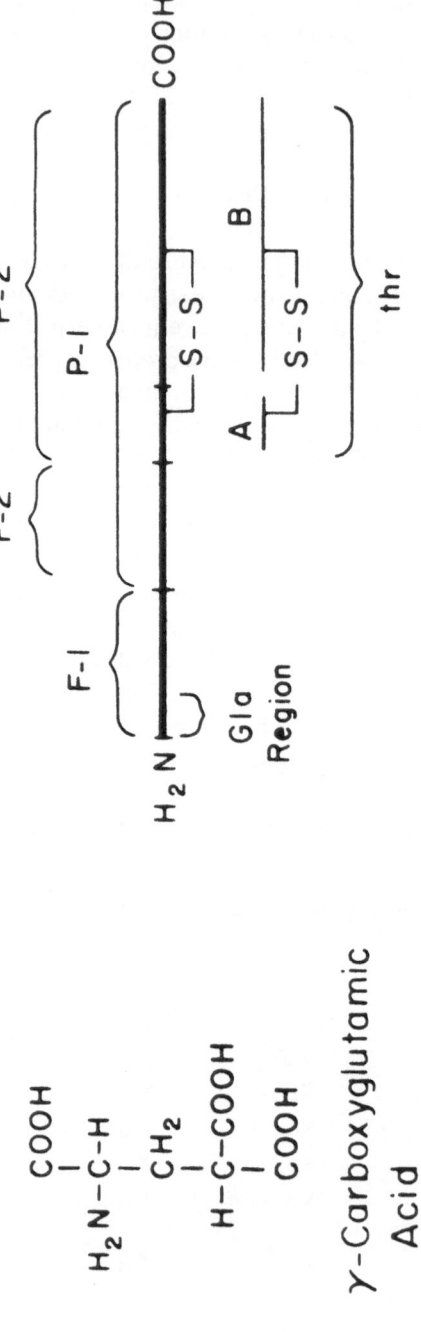

γ-Carboxyglutamic Acid

Ala-Asn-Lys-Gly-Phe-Leu-Gla-Gla-Val-Arg-Lys-Gly-Asn-Leu-Gla-Arg-Gla-Cys-Leu-

Gla-Gla-Pro-Cys-Ser-Arg-Gla-Gla-Ala-Phe-Gla-Ala-Leu-Gla-Ser-Leu-

Figure 12-3 γ-Carboxyglutamic acid (Gla) in the prothrombin molecule.

Which of these proteins is the physiologic precursor of prothrombin has not been determined.

Prothrombin Biosynthesis: Vitamin K-Dependent Carboxylation

After the vitamin K-dependent step in prothrombin synthesis was shown to be the formation of γ-carboxyglutamic acid residues, a system[11] previously shown to produce biologically active prothrombin was used to demonstrate that the addition of vitamin K and $H^{14}CO_3$ promoted the carboxylation of microsomal proteins (Figure 12-4). This carboxylation had essentially the same requirements[12] as the in vitro prothrombin-synthesizing system, and it was possible to show that the incorporated radioactivity was present as γ-carboxyglutamic acid residue in the fragment 1 region of prothrombin. These observations would appear to offer final proof of the role of vitamin K in the biosynthetic process.

The vitamin K-dependent carboxylase has been studied (see reference 1) in washed microsomes where the activity requires the presence of the precursor, O_2, vitamin K, and HCO_3^-, and is stimulated by an energy source. A stimulation of the system by the postmicrosomal supernatant can be replaced by the addition of NADH to the system, and this requirement has now been shown to be largely a requirement for the reduced form of vitamin K. We have now solubilized[13] the vitamin K-dependent carboxylase activity, and the solubilized preparation retains the basic requirement for reduced vitamin K and O_2 of the membrane-associated system, but is not inhibited by warfarin. Incubation of the solubilized system in the absence of ATP and in the presence of an ATP inhibitor does inhibit the membrane-bound (microsomal) carboxylase, but not the solubilized system. These data suggest that the energy to drive the reoxidation may come from the reoxidation of the reduced vitamin in the system. The currently established properties of the vitamin K-dependent carboxylase are presented in Table 12-2. Studies of the mechanism should be facilitated by the observation[14] that the pentapeptide Phe-Leu-Glu-Glu-Val will serve as a substrate for the carboxylase, and some idea of substrate specificity has been gained from a study of a number of synthetic peptides. These studies show that vitamin K functions to promote the carboxylation of a microsomal precursor to pro-thrombin, but does not establish its role in this reaction. There appear to be three generalized possibilities: 1) it may function to activate (or transfer) HCO_3^- (CO_2) for this carboxylation; 2) it may function to labilize the hydrogen at the γ-carboxyl of the precursor, so that it may accept the HCO_3^- (CO_2); or 3) it may function as an activator of one of the enzymes in this reaction (Figure 12-5). The latter possibility is probably least likely. A role of the vitamin as a membrane-associated, lipid-soluble CO_2 carrier is attractive, but there is no experimental evidence to support such a role.

138

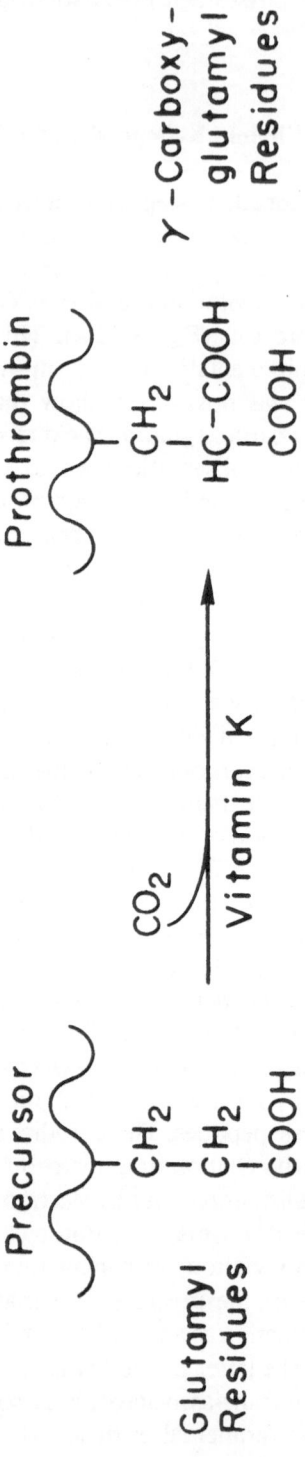

Figure 12-4 The effect of vitamin K on carboxylation of microsomal proteins.

Likewise, it seems possible that the reoxidation of the reduced form of the vitamin could be coupled to a labilization of a hydrogen on the γ-carbon of the glutamyl residues of the precursor to allow a direct attack of CO_2, but there is no experimental evidence to support this.

Table 12-2
Properties of the Vitamin K-Dependent Carboxylase

Absolute Requirements	Noninhibitory Conditions
Reduced vitamin K	ATP analog†
HCO_3^- (CO_2)	Avidin (biotin inhibitor)
Presence of precursor	EDTA
Known Inhibitors	Stimulatory Conditions
Chloro-K	Dithiothreitol
Warfarin*	Additional substrate (peptide)
p—Hydroxymercuribenzoate	
Spin-trapping agents	
(high concentration)	
Anaerobic conditions	

There is not complete agreement in the published literature on all points; the properties assigned represent the author's evaluation of the consensus of the published literature.
*Only when intact microsomes are present.
†Some inhibition when intact microsomes are present.

Mechanism of Coumarin Action

Numerous theories regarding the mechanism of action of the

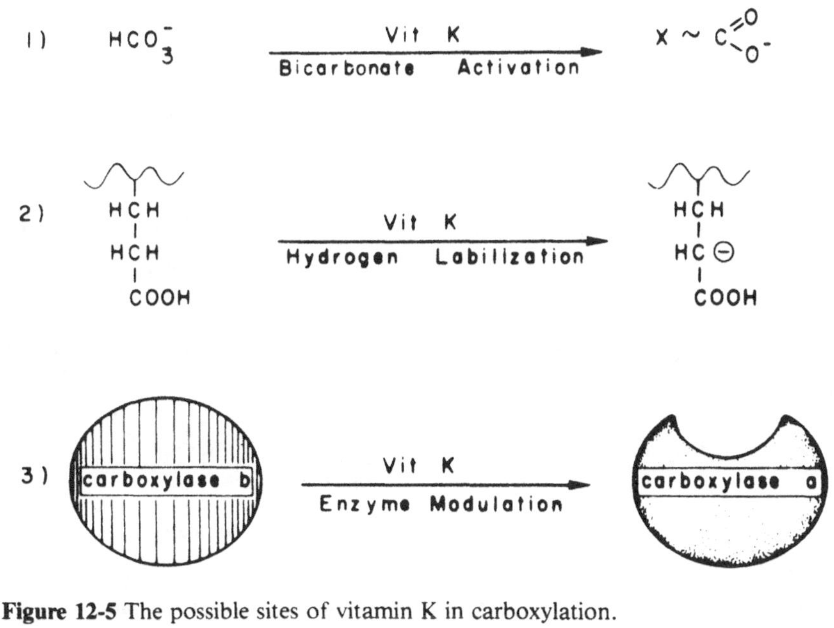

Figure 12-5 The possible sites of vitamin K in carboxylation.

140

coumarin anticoagulants have been proposed, but, without a clear understanding of the role of vitamin K, they have been difficult to test. Many workers in the past have assumed that the coumarin anticoagulants are direct antagonists of vitamin K at its active site (Figure 12-6A) or, more recently, that they act at a second site (Figure 12-6B) on the carboxylase system. It has also been postulated that coumarins act (Figure 12-6C) by blocking a normal transport route for the vitamin, rather than as inhibitors of the vitamin at its physiologically active site. At which membrane this warfarin-sensitive site functions or which cellular pools of the vitamin it separates is not defined by this theory. If the formation of the 2,3-epoxide of the vitamin (K-oxide) is involved in the action of the vitamin, the effect of coumarins might be exerted at this point (Figure 12-6D). It has been shown that warfarin blocks the action of the liver enzyme that reduces K-oxide to the vitamin; and if, as it has been suggested, the cyclic interconversion of the vitamin to its epoxide and then reduction to the vitamin form is required for its action, an inhibition of this cycle would result in an inhibition of the action of the vitamin.

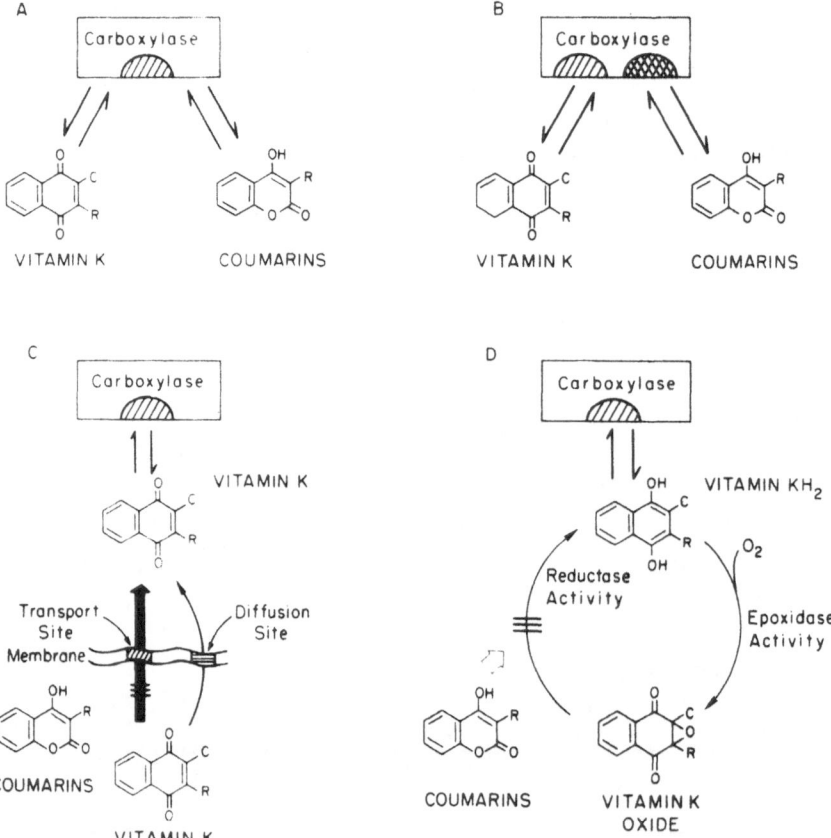

Figure 12-6 The possible sites of coumarin action in its antagonistic-vitamin K role.

Conclusion

During the last five years, our understanding of how vitamin K functions and of how vitamin K action is related to Ca⁺⁺ binding has developed from almost pure empiric description into a picture of biochemical processes at the molecular level. The basic mechanism of action of the vitamin K antagonist anticoagulants has been defined. The process by which vitamin K participation in protein carboxylation remains unknown, but it seems entirely possible that within a few more years the detailed mechanism of action of the vitamin will also be known. This will open opportunities for using this detailed knowledge of vitamin K action and anticoagulant action in developing more effective and safer anticoagulant therapies.

REFERENCES

1. Suttie JW, Jackson CM: Prothrombin structure, and biosynthesis. *Physiol Rev* 57:1-70, 1977.
2. Shah DV, Suttie JW: Mechanism of action of vitamin K: evidence for the conversion of a precursor protein to prothrombin in the rat. *Proc Nat Acad Sci USA* 68:1653-1657, 1971.
3. Garnot PO, Nilehn JE: Plasma prothrombin during treatment with Dicumarol. II. Demonstration of an abnormal prothrombin fraction. *Scand J Clin Lab Invest* 22:23-28, 1968.
4. Josso F, Lavergne JM, Gouault M, et al: Differents etats moleculaires du facter II (promthrombine). Leur etude a l'aide de la staphylocoagulase et d'anticorps anti-facteur II. I. Le facteur II chez les subjets traites par les antagonistes de la vitamine K. *Thromb Diath Haemorrh* 20:88-98, 1968.
5. Gitel SN, Owen WG, Esmon CT, et al: A polypeptide region of bovine prothrombin specific for binding to phospholipids. *Proc Nat Acad Sci USA* 70:1344-1348, 1973.
6. Stenflo J: Dicumarol-induced prothrombin in bovine plasma. *Acta Chem Scand* 24:3762-3763, 1970.
7. Stenflo J, Ferlund P, Egan W, et al: Vitamin K dependent modifications of glutamic acid residues in prothrombin. *Proc Natl Acad Sci USA* 71:2730-2733, 1974.
8. Nelsestuen GL, Zytkovicz TH, Howard JB: The mode of action of vitamin K. Identification of gamma-carboxyblutamic acid as a component of prothrombin. *J Biol Chem* 249:6347-6350, 1974.
9. Esmon CT, Grant GA, Suttie JW: Purification of an apparent rat liver prothrombin precursor: characterization and comparison to normal rat prothrombin. *Biochemistry* 14:1595-1600, 1975.
10. Grant GA, Suttie JW: Rat liver prothrombin precursors: purification of a second, more basic form. *Biochemistry* 15:5387-5393, 1976.
11. Shah DV, Suttie JW: The vitamin K dependent *in vitro* production of prothrombin. *Biochem Biophys Res Commun* 60:1397-1402, 1974.
12. Esmon CT, Sadowski JA, Suttie JW: A new carboxylation reaction. The vitamin K-dependent incorporation of H-14-CO3- into prothrombin. *J Biol Chem* 250:4744-4748, 1975.

13. Esmon CT, Suttie JW: Vitamin K-dependent carboxylase. Solubilization and properties. *J Biol Chem* 251:6238–6243, 1976.

14. Suttie JW, Hageman JM, Lehrman SR, et al: Vitamin K-dependent carboxylase. Development of a peptide substrate. *J Biol Chem* 251:5827–5830, 1976.

13 Surgical Approaches to Morbid Obesity

Baltej S. Maini, MD
George L. Blackburn, MD, PhD

The morbidly obese individual has been defined by Scott et al[1] as "one who has reached two or three or more times his ideal weight and who has maintained this level for five years or more despite efforts by himself, his family, and his physcian to bring about effective and sustained reduction of weight to acceptable medical standards." Morbid obesity has also been defined as "greater than 100 pounds over insurance table" ideal weight.[2] It is likely that operations designed to reduce weight in the morbidly obese individual will gradually assume increasing importance once the indications are better defined, further improvements in operative techniques are made, and the complications better understood and treated. The various surgical procedures currently being employed for the treatment of obesity will be reviewed and an analysis made of the complications.

HISTORICAL CONSIDERATIONS

The lack of adequate and long-term success in the control of morbid obesity by dietary regimens, behavior modification, and hypnosis led to the development of surgical procedures designed to create absorptive deficits by bypassing the small intestine. Subsequently, observations that patients with gastric resection remain thin contributed to the evolution of the gastric bypass operation designed to create a deficiency of intake. Kremen et al,[3] in 1954, described a patient in whom an end-to-end jejunoileostomy had been performed for the reduction of body weight. Nine years later, Payne[4] presented his results with 11 patients on whom jejunocolic shunts had been performed. The initial enthusiasm from the dramatic weight loss gradually waned, and although this procedure was originally designed to restore additional bowel length by a second operation, it was soon abandoned. The extreme morbidity with diarrhea, fluid and electrolyte disorders, and liver failure prevented continuation of the study. Modifications of this operation were adopted by Lewis et al[5,6] and later by Sherman et al.[7]

As more information and experience with various surgical procedures became available, the jejunoileal bypass assumed increasing importance in the management of patients with morbid obesity.[2,7-12] The applications of this operation to obese patients with hyperlipidemia became evident.[13,14] However, a certain degree of disenchantment with the intestinal bypass-related morbidity did persist, and procedures designed to limit the intake of food were designed. Gastroplasty was described by Printen and Mason,[15] to be abandoned soon by the authors because of poor results. Gastric bypass surgery soon evolved and seemed to be more effective in sustaining weight loss.[15-19]

INDICATIONS FOR THE SURGICAL THERAPY OF OBESITY

There is general agreement regarding the indications for surgical intervention in morbid obesity. It must be emphasized that prior to any patient's being considered for any form of therapy, a detailed metabolic work-up is necessary (Table 13-1). Surgical procedures must be performed at medical centers equipped for this type of work-up, and a metabolic follow-up is extremely important. The patient must be informed that the surgical procedures are of relatively recent origin and long-term effects of such operations are still largely unknown. In addition, the patient should become part of a study group, being made fully aware of the potential complications unique to these procedures.

The criteria for selection of patients must be adhered to rather strictly, both for optimizing results from surgery and also for proper follow-up and maintenance on dietary programs postoperatively. Table 13-2 lists the indications that are suggested.

The different surgical procedures for the control of morbid obesity will be reviewed, with special emphasis on technical considerations, complications, and associated systemic effects.

Table 13-1
Preoperative Evaluation of the Obese Patient

Complete blood count, Prothrombin time, Platelet count.

Serum chemistry: BUN, Glucose, Electrolytes, Calcium, Phosphate, Magnesium, Uric acid, Creatinine, Alkaline Phosphatase, SGOT, SGPT, LDH, CPK, Bilirubin, Total protein, Albumin/Globulin, Cholesterol.

Urinalysis, 24-hour urine urea nitrogen.

EKG, Chest x-ray.

Stool: 72-hour fecal fat and nitrogen.

Endocrine: Serum T4, Cortisol, Growth hormone, Glucose tolerance test, 24-hour urinary 17-ketosteroids and 17-ketogenic steroids.

Arterial blood gases.

Pulmonary function tests.

D-Xylose absorption test, Serum carotene, Vitamin B_{12}, Folate levels.

Bromsulphathalein retention.

Serum lipoprotein electrophoresis.

Total body^{40} K count.

Psychiatric evaluation.

Table 13-2
Patient Selection Criteria and Indications for Surgical Treatment of Morbid Obesity

Weight more than 100 lb (45 kg) over standard for height, sex, and age.

Failure of dietary control or inability to adhere to dietary methods.

Stable adult life pattern.

Presence of associated conditions:
Diabetes mellitus
Hypertension
Pickwickian syndrome
Congestive heart failure
Infertility
Degenerative arthritis (knees, hips)
Hyperlipidemia

Absence of:
Severe heart disease
Inflammatory bowel disease
Liver disease/cirrhosis/alcoholism
Renal failure

GENERAL CONSIDERATIONS

The preoperative work-up having been completed, it is occasionally necessary to bring the patients into the hospital for a period of diet control. With starvation, improved ventilatory function and reduction in arterial pCO_2 in patients with the Pickwickian syndrome have been reported.[20] This may facilitate the recovery of such patients from abdominal surgery, and postoperative maintenance on intravenous protein-sparing regimens[21,22] may have an additional role.

Whatever the choice of surgical procedure, preoperative parenteral antibiotic therapy is recommended, so as to attempt to minimize wound infection and related problems. A mechanical bowel preparation is necessary in patients with intestinal bypass procedures, and the addition of oral antibiotics to "sterilize" the gut is a matter of individual preference.

If cholelithiasis is coexistent (a high incidence is present in the obese individual[23]), cholecystectomy is carried out at the same time. Appendectomy is routinely performed. There is some argument regarding the routine employment of drains in the subcutaneous tissues; these can be used when deemed necessary by the operating surgeon. It will be interesting to watch the changing trends in the incidence of thrombophlebitis and pulmonary embolism, once the use of prophylactic low-dose heparin becomes widespread.[24]

Jejunocolic Bypass

This procedure was first performed by Payne.[4] Although the weight loss was impressive, intolerable metabolic problems (fluid and electrolyte disorders, dehydration, and liver failure) soon demonstrated the failure of this operation. There was a substantial incidence of reoperation for uncontrollable metabolic problems, and even death from liver failure occurred. This operation is mentioned only to prevent the evolution of the surgical approach to obesity. It is no longer performed.

Jejunoileal Bypass

Payne and DeWind[2] first published a report describing experiences with 58 patients undergoing an end-to-side jejunoileal bypass where 14 inches of jejunum was anastomosed to 4 inches of terminal ileum. An additional 12 patients had bypass procedures done with varying lengths of jejunum and ileum, but the 14-to-4 shunt gave the most acceptable results. A recent report by the same authors[10] describes their experience with 230 patients with this procedure.

End-to-side bypass Exposure is best obtained through a long transverse supraumbilical incision, with division of the rectus muscles. Liver biopsy is carried out routinely after exploration of the abdominal cavity. The ligament of Treitz is identified and the jejunum carefully measured along the mesenteric border and divided at the desired point. The proximal end of the bypassed jejunum is closed in two layers and fixed to the mesentery to avoid intussusception. The end of the proximal jejunum is anastomosed to the side of the ileum, 4 inches from the ileocecal valve or at any other predetermined site.

End-to-end bypass Sherman et al[7] proposed modifying the end-to-side technique because of some dissatisfaction arising from possible side effects (eg, weight gain or bacterial overgrowth in the bypassed segments) secondary to intestinal contents refluxing into the excluded intestine. Scott et al[25] have reviewed their experience with an operation in which 12 inches of jejunum are anastomosed end-to-end with 12 inches of ileum, utilizing a two-layer closure. Modifications of the bypass where 12 inches of jejunum are anastomosed to 8 or 6 inches of terminal ileum have also been used.[26] The proximal end of the bypassed jejunum is closed, while the distal end is anastomosed to the transverse colon. Buchwald et al[14] utilized an end-to-end anastomosis between 40 cm of jejunum and 4 cm of ileum, with drainage of the bypassed segment into the cecum. In a recent report, Benfield et al[11] described the anastomosis of 40 cm of jejunum to 10 cm of terminal ileum, with drainage of the bypassed segment into the transverse colon.

Postoperatively, patients may be kept in the intensive care unit when respiratory problems so dictate. However, a careful monitoring of arterial blood gases is indicated, and fluid and electrolyte balances are watched closely. Liver biopsies and biochemical monitoring of the liver function of those patients are carried out as suggested by individual protocols.

COMPLICATIONS

An excellent review of the surgical complications has been provided by Bray[27] and is depicted in Table 13-3. Caution must be exercised in choosing the operative procedure, since a shorter segment of intestine does result in a greater weight loss, but more nutritional problems as well.

Mortality Operative mortality has been attributed to a number of causes: liver failure, pulmonary embolism, cardiac failure, pancreatitis, hypocalcemia, sepsis, and wound dehiscence. While operative technique is obviously of critical importance in determining operative mortality, an adequate preoperative evaluation is emphasized. DeWind and Payne[10] have recently reported an 8% bypass-related incidence of death. In the patients who died, the mean initial weight (418 lb for men and 338 lb for women) was much higher than the entire group (mean 347 lb for men and 280 lb for

Table 13-3
Complications of Jejunoileostomy Used for Treatment of Obesity

Complications	Percent
Major	
Early	
Operative mortality	0–6.5
Pulmonary emboli	1–6
Wound infection	2–10
Gastrointestinal hemorrhage	0–6
Renal failure	0–9
Late	
Urinary calculi	3–30
Liver disease	0–14
Anemia	0–3
Acute cholecystitis	0–7
Intestinal obstruction	0–3.5
Minor	
Diarrhea	100
Minor electrolyte abnormalities	40–80
Hypoproteinemia	40–100
Vomiting	10–80
Polyarthritis	0–6
Hair loss	0–100

From Bray.[27] Adapted from material first published in *Nutrition in Disease,* Ross Laboratories, Columbus, Ohio, 1979.

women). Buchwald et al[14] have reported an operative mortality of 1%. It must be re-emphasized that only a well-trained team of physicians, psychologists, and surgeons working within the guidelines of clinical investigation should presently be carrying out this therapy.

Morbidity

Wound　Wound infection rates are not much different from those seen in surgical procedures involving the gut or biliary tract. Consideration must be given to the use of retention sutures in patients with coexistent chronic lung disease or other complications, although by and large the insertion of stay sutures is not a practical convenience.

Metabolic complications　Electrolyte problems following jejunoileal bypass are due to two factors: impaired absorptive capacity and rapid transit time. When the patient starts eating postoperatively, he may experience 8 to 20 liquid bowel movements per day, which gradually decrease to 4 to 10 semiformed stools per day. Hypokalemia, hyponatremia, dehydration, acidosis, hypocalcemia, and hypomagnesemia may occur, all of which can be life-threatening. Meticulous biochemical monitoring that includes the recording of stool and urine losses is required. At the time of discharge, patients should receive oral supplements of calcium and potassium, and an antidiarrheal agent. A tendency to a gradual lowering of serum calcium and potassium levels has been observed,[2,4,8] and routine supplementation is therefore recommended. This can gradually be tapered off when indicated, as the frequency of diarrhea and extent of electrolyte abnormalities decreases with time. Calcium can be provided easily by calcium antacids (eg, Tums and Titralac). Potassium is best provided by an effervescent liquid (eg, K-Lyte). Table 13-4 gives a list of high-potassium foods that are recommended in the postoperative period. Filtzer (personal communication) recommends the exteriorization of the proximal end of the bypassed segment and creation of a feeding jejunostomy for potassium and calcium supplements in instances where hypokalemia and hypocalcemia cannot be managed by routine oral supplementation. The jejunostomy tube can be withdrawn when the metabolic aberrations have been corrected and diarrhea controlled. The exteriorized segment can also be used for protein and calorie repletion if indicated, and for instillation of antibiotics when necessary.

Table 13-4
Foods with a High Potassium Content

Apricots, canned or dried	Juices
Artichoke	Nectarines
Asparagus, frozen	Oranges
Avocado	Parsnips
Bananas	Peaches, raw or dried
Blackberries, raw	Peas, dried split
Broccoli, fresh	Potatoes, sweet
Brussels sprouts	Potatoes, white
Cantaloupe	Pumpkin
Carrots, raw	Radishes
Cherries, raw	Soybeans
Cowpeas, cooked	Squash, winter
Grapes, raw	Strawberries, fresh

A reduction in total red blood cell count, especially in Pickwickian patients, has been reported.[4] By preserving the distal 12 inches of ileum, Scott et al[25] have obviated the need for supplementing vitamin B_{12} postoperatively, but weight loss may be reduced. A slow fall in serum protein levels, particularly albumin, also results.[2,4,28] In all likelihood this is largely related to a low protein intake; hence the need for diet containing adequate protein. Impairment of fat absorption has been demonstrated with relative uniformity in all series.[2,4,11,28] The amount of fat excreted can be directly correlated with the length of residual jejunum in continuity. Accompanying these effects, a

150

flattening of the glucose tolerance curve has been demonstrated. However, the D-Xylose absorption curve gradually resumes normalcy.[28,29]

Long-Term Effects   The severity of hair loss varies in different series, but occurs often enough to be noticed and is probably secondary to protein deficiency. Polyarthritis and polyarthralgia occur in about 10% of patients and, interestingly, in 19% of female patients reported by De-Wind and Payne.[10] The most frequent occurrence of arthritis is about three to six months after surgery and never severe enough to be crippling. No radiologic changes have been noted, and symptoms, if severe, usually subside with small doses of corticosteroids.

Calculi in the urinary tract, as an effect of jejunoileal bypass, are almost always composed of calcium oxalate. There is evidence to demonstrate an increased absorption of oxalate in these patients.[30] In addition, the hyperoxaluria may be related to an increased bile salt and glycine synthesis.[31] Table 13-5 lists many foods that are high in oxalate content; it may be beneficial to avoid them. An increased incidence of cholelithiasis has also been observed postoperatively.[12] A supersaturated bile resulting in a tendency to form gallstones has been detected in obese patients.[32] It is unclear whether this continues postoperatively, but an increase in bile salt synthesis secondary to excessive loss of bile salts in the feces is observed, with an increased glycine/taurine conjugation ratio in the lithogenic bile.[31]

Table 13-5
Foods with a High Oxalate Content

Almonds	Endive
Beans	Figs
Beet greens	Gooseberries
Beets	Okra
Cashew nuts	Plums
Chard	Raspberries
Chocolate	Rhubarb
Cocoa	Spinach
Concord grapes	Tea
Currants	Tomatoes

An interesting entity, "bypass enteritis," has been described by Passaro et al.[33] This occurs two to six weeks after bypass and ileosigmoidostomy, and results in fever, abdominal pain, diarrhea, and a tender abdomen. Radiologic examination shows distended bowel loops and/or free air in the peritoneal cavity. At celiotomy, pneumatosis cystoides intestinalis may be seen. A good response is obtained with intravenous antibiotics. This syndrome complex is, in all likelihood, related to overgrowth of enteric flora, particularly anaerobes. The presence of associated intestinal ileus acts as a contributing factor.

Colonic pseudo-obstruction can be seen occasionally after intestinal bypass operations, the site of pseudo-obstruction being determined by the point of drainage of the bypassed segment.[19] The symptoms are related to the increased population of obligate anaerobes. Conservative therapy with intravenous fluids, nasogastric suction, and antibiotic therapy is usually adequate. Palliative therapy with *Lactobacillus* may also be effective,[11] but if the problem is persistent, revision of the bypass may be necessary.

Another long-term effect is hepatic dysfunction. Approximately 50% of obese patients have abnormal liver histology, predominantly fatty metamorphosis, as described by Zelman.[34] Morbidly obese individuals, however, may show a fatty liver in about 75% of cases.[2,8,18] About 5% to 10% of patients may develop liver disease after intestinal bypass. The earliest manifestations are alterations in enzyme function, hepatomegaly, and hypoalbuminemia. Later, a rise in serum bilirubin occurs with progressive liver failure. Liver scans and liver biopsy can detect these changes early; hence the need for liver biopsy at six-month intervals until weight loss is stabilized for one year and until hepatic morphology has become normal or has remained stable.[19] In severe cases, cirrhosis, hepatic coma, ascites, and death may occur. The etiology of hepatic steatosis is unclear and may be related to a number of factors: 1)protein deficiency; 2) absorption of toxic bile acids (lithocholic acid and chenodeoxycholic acid); 3) absorption of bacterial toxins; 4)insult by alcohol ingestion (past or present); or 5) the length of the bypassed segment.

Early cases of hepatic dysfunction are easily treated by increasing oral protein intake. Patients with a more severe disorder need hospitalization and intravenous hyperalimentation, while a third group may require restoration of intestinal continuity to ensure survival. An interesting means of treating hepatic steatosis has been provided by Heimburger et al,[35] where treatment of fatty liver has been achieved by the administration of glucose-free amino acids. This encourages the mobilization of fat, while minimizing protein loss.[36] Liver failure is most often seen within the first year after surgery, and about 1% to 3% of all bypass patients succumb from this complication.

WEIGHT LOSS AFTER JEJUNOILEAL BYPASS

The degree of weight loss after jejunoileal bypass is dependent on several factors: 1) initial weight; 2) time between operation and evaluation, ie, duration of follow-up; and 3) the type of surgical procedure.

The maximum weight loss has been reported in the first year after operation[10,11] and may range between 30 and 150 lb. A gradual drop in weight continues up to the second year, after which there is a tendency for the weight to acquire a steady state. Although a positive correlation between initial weight and weight loss has been demonstrated by Benfield et al[11] and Backman,[37] the same observation has not been made by DeWind and Payne.[10]

Several investigators undertook to perform the end-to-end bypass as opposed to the end-to-side bypass, as a result of the observation that weight loss levelled off after about one year and, in some instances, a gain in weight occurred. Buchwald and Varco[13] and Scott et al[1,38] reported an improvement in the results with an end-to-end bypass. A study by Benfield et al[11] showed a slightly greater weight loss in the group of patients with an end-to-end anastomosis as compared to the patients with an end-to-side bypass, but the results were not statistically significant.

Finally, an analysis of the length of intestine in continuity shows that operations with more than 25 inches (64 cm) of intestine produce very little weight loss, as demonstrated by Weismann.[39]

The changes in body composition after intestinal bypass surgery have been studied.[26,40] Prior to surgery, patients have 60% to 65% excess body fat, acccompanied by an excessive (21%) hydration of lean tissues. After surgery, a loss of fat mass is observed, accompanied by a reduction in total body water. Analysis of lean body mass (LBM) (derived from total body [40]K counts) shows an initial loss, but a reasonable maintenance of LBM in view of fat reduction and a lower level of hydration of lean tissues. In the first six months after intestinal bypass surgery, a 25% loss of LBM, which is about 50% of total weight loss, is observed. This is a significant depletion of lean tissue, and is not entirely desirable. An improved body composition in the group of patients undergoing end-to-end anastomosis as compared to the end-to-side group has been suggested.

GASTRIC BYPASS

This operation is designed to limit the intake of food, and intestinal absorption and digestion remain unaffected.

The abdomen is best approached by a bilateral subcostal incision, but an upper midline incision is preferred by some surgeons. It is necessary to carefully identify and divide the short gastric vessels so as to preserve the spleen. The left gastric vessels are identified and branches to the lesser curvature are divided close to the stomach, in order not to compromise the circulation to the gastric remnant. The stomach is divided, leaving about 10% of the stomach to form the pouch. The distal segment is closed in two layers; a stapling device may be used if desired. The medial portion of the gastric stump is closed in two layers, and a 2-cm area is left at the lateral margin for anastomotic purposes. A retrocolic anastomosis with the jejunum is carried out, forming a gastroenterostomy with a 12-mm diameter. Since enough mobility of the stomach has been obtained by dividing the short gastric vessels, the stomach is anchored to the transverse mesocolon, thereby obviating any efferent or afferent loop obstruction. The bypassed segment (90% of the intact stomach) is sutured to the anterior surface of the upper 10%; this prevents torsion or stasis in the remnant. Closure of the abdomen is effected in layers and intraabdominal drains are not necessary.

Postoperatively the patient is maintained on nasogastric suction, and oral feedings are resumed when indicated by clinical assessment.

Complications

Early   Anastomotic leaks occur because of a compromised circulation to the gastric pouch. It is important to divide the branches of the left gastric artery immediately adjacent to the lesser curvature. If the left gastric artery is tied close to its origin from the celiac axis, ischemia of the fundic segment results, since the short gastric vessels have also been divided. If the left gastric artery is divided just distal to the takeoff of the ascending esophageal artery, the latter may be the only blood vessel supplying the gastric pouch. These factors coupled with edema in Hofmeister's pouch may further contribute to ischemia at the gastroenterostomy site.

Problems of wound infection, dehiscence, and pulmonary embolism are no different than those described with the intestinal bypass procedures. Persistent vomiting, which is a frequent occurrence in these patients, can be severe enough to cause electrolyte disturbances. If vomiting is secondary to stomal dysfunction, it can be treated easily with nasogastric suction and intravenous fluids. On most occasions, however, vomiting is secondary to eating rapidly and too much. Vigorous control of eating habits is essential to avoid this problem.

Printen and Mason[15] showed an early mortality of 4.6%. Mason et al reported a 3% early mortality in 442 patients undergoing gastric bypass.[17]

Late   Of patients undergoing gastric bypass, 1.8% will develop stomal ulceration.[17] Anemia is an early indicator of stomal ulcer and, when present, must be investigated by endoscopy. If medical therapy is unsuccessful, vagotomy is necessary. The low incidence of stomal ulceration rests on the fact that a small fundic pouch has fewer parietal cells, and so less acid secretion from the stomach bathes the jejunum. But more important is the observation that the constant flow of acid from the excluded gastric segment into the duodenum inhibits gastrin release and maintains the acid secretion at a low level.[41] In addition, it is conceivable that less acid is secreted by the antrum, since as a result of the bypass there is no stimulus by distension with food. Further long-term follow-up, however, is still necessary to evaluate this potential problem.

Weight Loss in Gastric Bypass

In the series of Mason et al[17] the average weight loss at 1, 2, 3, and 5 years remains about 36 kg. About one-third of the patients can be expected to lose 50 kg at the end of 3 years. A revision of the stoma (from 12 mm to 9 mm) is necesssary in about 11% of patients, and a second revision may occasionally be essential to produce adequate weight loss.

Upon review of the data available on the gastric bypass procedure, and from our own experience, it is evident that although the gastric bypass may take a longer operating time and the degree of weight loss may not parallel that seen in jejunoileal bypass, the advantages are numerous. Nutritional, metabolic, electrolytic, hepatic, and other systemic problems do not exist with the gastric bypass procedure. The morbidity is significantly lower, and the eating habits are self-limiting: excessive carbohydrates cause dumping, and a large volume of food makes these patients vomit. Dietary surveillance does not end after surgery in gastric bypass; strict monitoring is often necessary.

An initial appraisal of ^{40}K counting in obese patients after gastric bypass surgery reveals that weight loss consists largely of fat, and lean body mass is minimally depleted (Table 13-6). Weight loss as measured by reduction of fat mass may approach the maximum possible loss of 0.25 kg/day as suggested by Yang and Van Itallie.[42] This is an encouraging observation, and long-term follow-up is currently under way. This is in direct contrast to the changes after jejunoileal bypass, where 50% of weight loss in the first six months after surgery consists of lean tissue. Although weight loss with the gastric bypass is less than that seen with jejunoileal bypass, the amount of fat loss appears to be identical. The excess weight loss in intestinal bypass is secondary to associated depletion of lean tissue, and this is a metabolically undesirable effect.

Table 13-6
Changes in Body Composition After Gastric Bypass

	Preoperative	Postoperative (mo)			
		2	4	8	14
Weight (kg)					
Patient 1	132.68	115.55	108.52	81.19	65.10
Patient 2	176.68		146.85	138.51	
Total body ^{40}K (g)					
Patient 1	102	83	87	94	95
Patient 2	167		159	153	
LBM (kg)					
Patient 1	39.60	32.23	33.78	36.50	36.89
Patient 2	61.14		58.21	56.01	
LBM as % of weight					
Patient 1	29.85	27.89	31.13	44.95	56.67
Patient 2	34.60		39.64	40.94	

CONCLUSIONS

There is little doubt that having fulfilled the criteria for operative intervention, surgical treatment is justified and necessary in morbidly obese patients. Nevertheless, operations for this malady are still investigational, and accurate follow-up data must continually be made available. The operative procedures should provide an adequate amount of weight loss (and thus protection from the deleterious systemic effects of obesity), but at the same time prevent nutritional and metabolic compromise.

REFERENCES

1. Scott HW Jr, Law DH IV, Sandstead HH, et al: Jejunoileal shunt in surgical treatment of morbid obesity. *Ann Surg* 171: 770, 1970.
2. Payne JH, DeWind LT: Surgical treatment of obesity. *Am J Surg* 118: 141, 1969.
3. Kremen AJ, Linner JH, Nelson C: An experimental evaluation of the nutritional importance of proximal and distal small intestine. *Ann Surg* 140: 439, 1954.
4. Payne JH: Metabolic observations in patients with jejunocolic shunts. *Am J Surg* 106:273, 1963.
5. Lewis LA, Turnbull RB, Page IH: "Short circuiting" of the small intestine. *JAMA* 182: 77, 1962.
6. Lewis LA, Turnbull RB, Page IH: Effects of jejunocolic shunt on obesity, serum lipoproteins, lipids and electrolytes. *Arch Intern Med* 117: 4, 1966.
7. Sherman CD Jr. May AG, Nye W, et al: Clinical and metabolic studies following bowel bypassing for obesity. *Ann NY Acad Sci* 131:614, 1965.
8. Salmon PA: The results of small intestinal bypass operations for the treatment of obesity. *Surg Gynecol Obstet* 132: 965, 1971.
9. Schwartz MZ, Varco RL, Buchwald H: Preoperative preparation, operative technique and postoperative care of patients undergoing jejunoileal bypass for massive exogenous obesity. *J Surg Res* 14: 147, 1973.
10. DeWind LT, Payne HJ: Intestinal bypass surgery for morbid obesity. *JAMA* 236: 2298, 1976.
11. Benfield JR, Greenway FL, Bray GA, et al: Experience with jejunoileal bypass for obesity. *Surg Gynecol Obstet* 143: 401, 1976.
12. Payne JH, DeWind L, Schwab CE, et al: Surgical treatment of morbid obesity. *Arch Surg* 106: 432, 1973.
13. Buchwald H, Varco RL: A bypass operation for obese hyperlipidemics. *Surgery* 70: 62, 1970.
14. Buchwald H, Varco RL, Moore RB, et al: Intestinal bypass procedures. *Curr Probl Surg* April, 1975.
15. Printen KJ, Mason EE: Gastric surgery for relief of morbid obesity. *Arch Surg* 106: 428, 1973.
16. Mason EE, Ito C: Gastric bypass. *Ann Surg* 170: 329, 1969.
17. Mason EE, Printen KJ, Hartford CE, et al: Optimizing results of gastric bypass. *Ann Surg* 182: 405, 1975.
18. Soper RT, Mason EE, Printen KJ, et al: Gastric bypass for morbid obesity in children and adolescents. *J Pediatr Surg* 10: 51, 1975.
19. Bray GA, Barry RE, Benfield JR, et al: Intestinal bypass operation as a treatment of obesity. *Ann Intern Med* 85: 97, 1976.

20. Fried PI, McClean PA, Phillipson EA, et al: Effect of ketosis on respiratory sensitivity to carbon dioxide in obesity. *N Engl J Med* 294: 1081, 1976.

21. Freeman JB, Stegink LD, Meyer D, et al: Metabolic effects of amino acid vs. dextrose infusions in surgical patients. *Arch Surg* 110: 916, 1975.

22. Blackburn GL, Bistrian BR: Surgical technique in the treatment of adolescent obesity, in Collip PJ (ed): *Childhood Obesity*, Acton, Mass, Publishers Science Group, 1975.

23. Marks HH: Influence of obesity on morbidity and mortality. *Bull NY Acad Med* 36: 296, 1960.

24. Tice DA: Low dosage of heparin. *Surg Gynecol Obstet* 143: 970, 1976.

25. Scott HW Jr, Sandstead HH, Brill AG, et al: Experience with a new technique of intestinal bypass in the treatment of morbid obesity. *Ann Surg* 174: 560, 1971.

26. Brill AB, Sandstead HH, Price R, et al: Changes in body composition after jejunoileal bypass in morbidly obese patients. *Am J Surg* 123: 49, 1973.

27. Bray GA: *The Obese Patient*. Philadelphia, WB Saunders Co, 1976.

28. Shibata HR, MacKenzie JR, Long RC: Metabolic effects of controlled jejunocolic bypass. *Arch Surg* 95: 413, 1967.

29. Scott HW Jr, Law DH IV: Clinical appraisal of jejunoileal shunt in patients with morbid obesity. *Am J Surg* 171: 246, 1969.

30. Earnest DL, Williams HE, Admirand WH: Excessive absorption of oxalates contributes to hyperoxaluria in patients with ileal disease. *Gastroenterology* 64: A40, 1973.

31. Wise L, Stein T: Biliary and urinary calculi. Pathogenesis following small bowel bypass for obesity. *Arch Surg* 110: 1043, 1975.

32. Freeman JB, Meyer PB, Printen KB, et al: Analysis of gallbladder bile in morbid obesity. *Am J Surg* 131: 169, 1976.

33. Passaro E Jr, Drenick E, Wilson SE: Bypass enteritis. A new complication of jejunoileal bypass for obesity. *Am J Surg* 131: 169, 1976.

34. Zelman S: The liver in obesity. *Arch Intern Med* 90: 141, 1952.

35. Heimburger SL, Steiger E, Logerfo P, et al: Reversal of severe fatty hepatic infiltration after intestinal bypass for morbid obesity by calorie-free amino acid infusion. *Am J Surg* 129: 229, 1975.

36. Blackburn GL, Flatt JP, Hensle TW: Peripheral amino acid infusions, in Fischer J (ed): *Total Parenteral Nutrition*, Boston, Little Brown Company, 1976.

37. Backman L: The rate of weight loss after intestinal bypass operations for obesity: an analysis of factors of significance. *Acta Chir Scand* 141: 424, 1975.

38. Scott HW Jr, Dean R, Shull HJ: New considerations in use of jejunoileal bypass in patients with morbid obesity. *Ann Surg* 177: 723, 1973.

39. Weismann RE: Surgical palliation of massive and severe obesity. *Am J Surg* 125: 437, 1973.

40. Scott HW Jr, Brill AB, Price R: Body composition in morbidly obese patients before and after jejunoileal bypass. *Ann Surg* 182: 395, 1975.

41. Mason EE, Ito C: Gastric bypass in obesity. *Surg Clin North Am* 47: 1345, 1967.

42. Yang MU, Van Itallie TB: Composition of weight loss during short-term weight reduction. Metabolic response to starvation and low-calorie ketogenic and non-ketogenic diets. *J Clin Invest* 58: 722, 1976.

14 The Fetal Alcohol Syndrome

Eileen Ouellette, MD

The term "fetal alcohol syndrome" has been introduced to describe a number of features seen in some children born to mothers who have drunk large amounts of alcohol chronically before and during pregnancy. The constellation of features seen in these children consists of prenatal and postnatal growth retardation, developmental delay, mental retardation, and a number of major and minor congenital anomalies. (Table 14-1).

Developmental defects of the brain, microcephaly, and a variety of congenital heart disorders have been among the major defects noted. Minor facial anomalies have been descibed by a number of authors who have emphasized the presence of short palpebral fissures, epicanthal folds, ptosis, abnormal upper lip, abnormally formed ears, micrognathia, and cleft palate. Other congenital malformations reported have included congenital hip dislocation, limitation of elbow extension, altered palmar creases, and phalangeal anomalies. In some cases, anomalous external genitalia, capillary hemangiomas, extra nipples, and skeletal and renal anomalies have been found. Neural tube defects have recently been reported.

Some researchers estimate that the frequency of alcohol embryopathy is as common as 1 or 2 per 1000 live births for the full constellation of features, with the frequency of partial expression at possibly 3 to 5 per 1000

157

Table 14-1
Abnormalities Associated with Fetal Alcohol Syndrome

Craniofacial Anomalies
  Microcephaly
  Eye abnormalities
    Epicanthal folds
    Telecanthus
    Short palpebral fissures
    Corneal opacity
    Ptosis
    High myopia
    Strabismus
    Tortuosity of retinal vessels
  Flattened nasal bridge
  Abnormally formed ears
  Maxillary hypoplasia
  Narrow vermilion border of upper lip
  Small mandible
  Cleft palate

Joint and Limb Malformations
  Limitation of elbow extension
  Phalangeal anomalies
    Small nails
    Clinodactyly
  Abnormal palmar creases
  Dislocated hips

Cardiac Abnormalities
  Atrial septal defects
  Ventricular septal defects
  Tetralogy of Fallot
  Patent ductus arteriosus
  Aortic arch interruption type A
  Peripheral pulmonic stenosis

Growth Abnormalities
  Prematurity
  Intrauterine growth retardation
  Postnatal growth retardation
    Short stature
    Diminished weight

Renal Anomalies
  Hydronephrosis
  Single kidney
  Hypoplastic kidneys

Functional Abnormalities
  Neonatal
    Poor suck
    Hypotonia
    Tremulousness
  Postnatal
    Developmental delay
    Mental retardation
    Poor gross motor coordination
    Poor fine motor coordination

Other Findings
  Hydrocephalus
  Neural tube defects
  Single umbilical artery
  Noonan's syndrome
  Klippel-Feil syndrome
  Capillary hemangiomas
  Abnormal external genitalia
  Accessory nipples
  Adrenal cortical carcinoma
  Spastic diplegia

live births. The risk of producing an abnormal child for a mother with alcohol abuse is unknown.

Information is still lacking concerning the full scope and gravity of the deleterious effects on the fetus of chronic maternal alcohol abuse prior to and during pregnancy. Effects produced range from mildly impaired to profoundly afflicted children, and some fatalities have been reported.

It is unknown how many children's lives have been permanently afflicted by excessive alcohol use in their mothers.

Historical Review

The belief that parental alcohol intake may be injurious to the fetus dates back to antiquity. The Greek god Hephaestus was believed by some to be deformed because his parents, Zeus and Hera, were intoxicated at the time of his conception. Ancient Sparta and Carthage passed laws prohibiting the use of alcohol by newly married couples on their wedding night so that defective children would not be conceived. Plato recommended that newly married couples not use alcohol. In a statement attributed to Aristotle, "Foolish and drunken and harebrained women most often bring forth children like unto themselves, morose and languid."

Biblical references also contain warnings against parental drinking. In Judges 13:3-4, an angel appears to Samson's mother saying, "Thou art barren, and without children, but thou shalt conceive, and bear a son. Now therefore beware, and drink not wine nor strong drink, and eat not any unclean thing."

Throughout the Middle Ages the belief that parental intoxication at the time of conception could produce abnormal offspring flourished. Alcohol consumption during these years was primarily in the form of wine, beer, ale, and cider. Little is known of the magnitude of the problem of alcoholism at that time.

By the early 18th century, distilled spirits became readily available in Western Europe. From 1720 to 1750 the so-called gin epidemic created a social crisis in England. In an effort to help rich landowners, legislation was passed lifting traditional restrictions on the distillation of spirits, and cheap, plentiful gin became available.

The College of Physicians petitioned Parliament in 1726 for control of distillation, citing gin as "a cause of weak, feeble and distempered children." In 1736, a committee of the Middlesex Sessions wrote, "Unhappy mothers habituate themselves...children are born weak and sickly, and often look shriveled and old as though they had numbered many years."

Renewed concerns about the harmful effects of excessive alcohol use on offspring occurred. Henry Fielding wrote in 1751, "What must become an infant who is conceived in *Gin*? with the poisonous Distillations of which it is nourished, both in the Womb and at the Breast." The famous etching "Gin Lane" by William Hogarth was published in 1751. This not only illustrated the social disorganization brought on by excessive alcohol intake, but stressed in its central figure the effects of maternal drinking on a child. In 1751, Parliament reinstituted controls over the manufacture of distilled spirits. Further descriptions continued to appear, citing early death, feeblemindedness, and epilepsy in offspring of drunken parents throughout the remainder of the century.

America did not have a gin epidemic during the 18th century and little interest was evidenced on the effects of alcohol. Benjamin Rush, a signer of the Declaration of Independence and one of the most significant early American physicians, attacked misconceptions about alcohol at the end of the 18th century. He was the first English-speaking physician to propose that alcoholism was a disease. However, he also believed that pregnancy was a disease. He wrote that the condition of the parents at the time of conception would determine the child's constitution, and that all of these characteristics were inherited. In 1787, he warned against prescribing alcohol to pregnant women because of its potential production of dependence.

In 1813, Thomas Trotter expressed concern about the birth of "puny" children as a result of alcoholism in either parent, basing his concerns on the theory that alcohol would injure the sex organs, thus producing diseased offspring. Parliament commissioned a Select Committee on Drunkenness that reported in 1834 to the House of Commons that infants of alcoholic mothers had "a starved, shriveled and imperfect look." Charles Dickens was aware of these medical reports. In *Pickwick Papers*, he referred to a character, Betsy Martin, as having one eye because her mother drank bottled stout.

With the growth of the temperance movement, further constraints against women ingesting alcohol when pregnant appeared. Arrest of growth and destruction of the health of the infant were cited in 1837 by Ryan, but Forbes in 1848 advised alcohol as beneficial for pregnant and lactating women with congestive problems.

Samuel Gridley Howe performed the first piece of epidemiologic research on the topic of parental drinking in 1848 when he reported to the Legislature of Massachusetts after having examined the family histories of 300 institutionalized idiots. One hundred forty-five had alcoholic parents. A second epidemiologic study was carried out in Switzerland by Bezzola between 1880 and 1890, in which he found that there was an increase in the birth of idiots nine months after wine festivals, with a corresponding drop in normal births.

The theory of the inheritance of alcoholism from parent to child has been prominent. Robert Burton's *Anatomy of Melancholy* published in 1621 cited Plutarch: "One drunkard begets another." Sir Francis Galton in 1889 first spoke against the concept of inheritance of these abnormal children, emphasizing that while the alcoholic woman's tissues are soaked in alcohol, the unborn infant must also be alcoholized. He also suggested that alcohol must be ingested postnatally in the mother's milk.

Sullivan studied maternal alcoholism during pregnancy in the late 19th century. In 1899 he reported on 120 female alcoholics at the Liverpool jail. They were screened to exclude those with histories of syphilis, tuberculosis, and degenerative disease. Of 600 children born to these women, only 44% lived longer than two years. The remainder died before that age or were stillborn. Sullivan also studied 28 female relatives of a study group, who did not show alcohol abuse. Only 24% of their offspring died by two years. In addition to this 2.5 × increase in the death rate among children of alcoholic women, he found that the death rate increased with increasing parity. In this study Sullivan also obtained data on fathers' drinking habits and excluded these as unrelated to the infant death rate in children of alcoholic mothers. The main cause of death of children in Sullivan's series was epilepsy.

A number of anecdotal reports or poorly controlled studies continued to appear in the late 19th and early 20th centuries, all citing the potential for damage in offspring of alcoholic parents.

Theories of the way in which alcohol affected offspring fell into two groups: one group put forth the blastophthoric theory that alcohol affected the generative organs, thereby producing diseased offspring; the other stressed the transmission of alcohol via the placenta and/or mother's milk into the offspring and suggested an acquired origin.

The hereditary infant alcoholics were said to be feeble, susceptible to infection, and likely to die in infancy. They sometimes showed tremor. If they lived, they were said to be more susceptible to medical illness, epilepsy, and chorea. Acquired infant alcoholics were those who became addicted to alcohol by ingesting mother's milk or alcohol-based medicines. They were described as showing restlessness, tremor, and seizures.

When prohibition came into effect in the United States in 1919, articles concerning alcohol and pregnancy abruptly disappeared. Beliefs in the hazards of maternal alcohol abuse in pregnancy fell into disrepute.

In 1942, Haggard and Jellinek[1] firmly stated that, "No acceptable evidence has ever been offered to show that acute alcoholic intoxication has any effect whatsoever on the human germ, or has any influence in altering heredity, or is the cause of any abnormality in the child." They cited poor nutrition in the mother and environmental disorder in the home as causes of the symptoms seen in children. This was refuted 18 years later by Christiaens et al[2] who described morphologic abnormalities in offspring of alcoholic parents. Sandberg noted in 1961[3] that infants of alcoholic mothers showed withdrawal symptoms similar to those produced with narcotics. Schaeffer cited a similar case in 1962.[4]

The pioneer modern work on the prenatal effects of alcohol was carried out by Lemoine et al in Marseilles in 1968.[5] They studied 127 offspring of alcoholic parents and described morphologic abnormalities that included low birth weight, short stature, delayed growth and development, craniofacial and cardiac abnormalities, retarded intellectual and motor development, and impaired school function. In the United States, Ulleland[7] reported that 10 of 12 children born to 11 female alcoholics were small for gestational age. Development was found to be retarded or borderline even when corrected for prematurity. Postnatal growth retardation occurred.

In subsequent papers, Jones et al[8-11] retrospectively examined eight unrelated children born to chronically alcoholic mothers and described the growth, morphologic, and developmental abnormalities for which they subsequently coined the term "the fetal alcohol syndrome."

Women and Alcohol

Studies of alcohol intake among women are of recent origin, and significant differences are reported between male and female alcoholics. Women tend to be more solitary in their drinking patterns and alcohol intake is reported to increase in the immediate premenstrual period.

Heavy-drinking women are said to have more marital problems than heavy-drinking men, and are often from families in which a controlling mother and a passive alcoholic father were present during their formative years.

Alcohol abuse plays a significant role in inadequate mothering and in the production of child abuse and incest. Some series report intoxication in up to 50% of batterers.

Drinking among American women has been rising steadily since World War II, and now constitutes a major public health problem.[12] Estimates of the number of female alcoholics in the United States range from 700,000 to 4,500,000. A particular concern is that excessive drinking is rising at a rapid rate. The highest proportion of heavy drinkers among women is between the ages of 21 and 29, the age of peak reproductive years.

A national survey[13] of students done in 1974 indicates that among seventh graders, 63% of boys and 54% of girls have had a drink. This proportion of teenage drinkers increases with each grade to 93% of 12th grade boys and 87% of 12th grade girls.

The use of alcohol among girls and among women is approaching that of boys and men. Reliable data concerning alcoholism in women are difficult to obtain as the female alcoholic has a greater tendency to drink secretly in the privacy of her home and therefore comes to professional attention later than the male alcoholic, who often is identified through poor work performance or automobile accidents.

Recent studies show that all women tend to decrease their alcoholic intake during the early months of pregnancy, presumably from a combination of factors. The nausea and vomiting of early pregnancy with the production of gastric distress have been cited as causes for the decreased desire for alcoholic beverages at that time. Motivation for providing a maximum nurturing environment for the fetus may also be a contributing factor.

In a study of 633 heavy-drinking women of low socioeconomic class in an inner-city ghetto environment,[14] we found a significant decrease in the amount of alcohol consumed by heavy-drinking women during the early months of pregnancy. Heavy-drinking women were defined by the criteria of Cahalan, Crisin, and Crossley[15] and include those women who drink five or more drinks on one occasion and who consume the equivalent of a consistent average of at least 135 ml of absolute alcohol per day. We found that women during this time were quite responsive to therapeutic intervention and many women omitted alcohol throughout the rest of their pregnancy as a result of the counseling provided.

In another study of 41 predominantly white, middle-class alcoholic women in their early 30s, Little and Streissguth[16] found that while overall alcohol consumption decreased during pregnancy, the number of days of binge drinking increased. Women were defined as alcoholic if they "reported a major drinking problem before pregnancy or consumed an average of at least the equivalent of 3 oz of ethanol daily in the year prior to conception." A binge was defined as 1 day or more when drinking was at least double the regular level and a minimum of 3 oz of absolute alcohol was consumed. The authors required that binges be separated by at least 10 days and comprise no more than 7 days each month.

Measurement of alcohol intake   Numerous scales exist to measure alcohol consumption; none is perfect. Cahalan et al[15] have devised a Volume-Variability Index (VVI) that measures the average daily volume of alcohol consumed and also measures the variability of alcohol intake according to the number of drinks consumed. This formula enables one to observe the pattern of drinking more specifically.

Another form of measurement, also devised by Cahalan et al,[15] measures the quantity, frequency, and variability of alcohol consumption and is called "QFV Index." This calculation reflects the quantity and variability of consumption of the most frequently consumed beverages combined with the frequency of drinking any alcoholic beverage. A modification of this method calculates separate QFV scores for wine, beer, and distilled spirits.

It is important when assessing data on the impact of alcohol consumption during pregnancy that very detailed intake information be obtained, and some standard measurement of alcohol intake be calculated.

Criteria for the diagnosis of alcoholism   Among the early signs of alcohol abuse are flushed face, tachycardia, chronic gastritis, gulping drinks or surreptitious drinking, increased absence from work for a variety of reasons, loss of interest in activities not directly associated with drinking, unexpected changes in family, social, and business relationships, job loss due to interpersonal difficulties, separation, and divorce.

Characteristics of the middle stage of alcoholism are vascular engorgement of the face, increased incidence of infections, cardiac arrhythmias, peripheral neuropathy, ecchymoses or burns on limbs or chest, and drinking to relieve anger, insomnia, fatigue, depression, or social discomfort.

Serious medical signs and symptoms are present during the last stages of alcoholism. Tremor, withdrawal seizures, delirium tremens, Wernicke's syndrome, Korsakoff's syndrome, Laënnec's cirrhosis, pancreatitis, anemia and clotting disorders, cerebellar degeneration, and cardiomyopathy may be present. The individual may seek employment that facilitates drinking, have frequent automobile accidents and frequent changes of residence for poorly defined reasons, make numerous inappropriate telephone calls, have outbursts of rage, and may make suicidal gestures while drinking.

Shaw and Leiber[17] have reported that alterations in the plasma α-amino-n-butyric acid/leucine ratio occur in alcoholics and can act as an empiric biochemical marker for the disorder. Where doubt concerning the diagnosis occurs in the physician's mind, this blood test may be helpful.

Ethanol Metabolism in Humans and Animals

Ethanol is a small molecule as compared with other psychoactive drugs. It is rapidly absorbed through the mucosal membranes of the gastrointestinal tract, especially the duodenum and jejunum, and enters the portal circulation. It can also be absorbed through the respiratory tract. It is rapidly distributed throughout the body and diffuses across capillary and tissue membranes by simple diffusion. Within a few minutes after oral ingestion, it has been circulated to every tissue in the body. It is blocked by the blood-brain barrier and also passes readily through the placenta into the fetus.

As it passes through the individual cell membrane, the alcohol molecule affects the stabilization of the membrane. Inside the cell, the molecule also affects the membrane permeability and its transport mechanism. In the cytoplasm, changes are effected in the intracellular enzyme systems, mitochondria, and endoplasmic reticulum.

Ethanol is broken down by alcohol dehydrogenase. One of its metabolic breakdown products is acetaldehyde. Alcohol dehydrogenase activity has been detected in 2-month-old human fetuses, although it is only approximately 3% to 4% of adult activity at that time. Activity of this enzyme in the adult range is found after 5 years of age. Microsomal ethanol-oxidizing enzymes and catalases have also been measured in utero.

In utero effects   Alcohol passes rapidly from the maternal circulation to the fetus and assumes approximately the same concentration as in maternal blood. Alcohol levels within the fetal circulation fall more slowly than in the maternal circulation, so that detectable levels of alcohol are still present in the fetus after the alcohol has been totally cleared from the maternal circulation. Not only does alcohol enter the fetal circulation but it is excreted into the amniotic fluid where it remains in essentially the same concentration for several hours until it is cleared slowly. Changes are seen in fetal acid-base balance, cerebral function, and metabolism. Serious maternal illnesses have been described from alcohol abuse in pregnancy, including alcoholic ketoacidosis and cirrhosis.

Postnatal effects   Ethanol and acetaldehyde levels have been measured in the peripheral blood and milk of lactating women and animals. Ethanol has been found to reach human milk in a concentration similar to that in peripheral maternal blood, decreasing with decreasing ethanol content of the blood, but acetaldehyde has not been detected in milk, even in the presence of considerable amounts in the blood.

Clinical Effects of Maternal Alcohol Abuse on Offspring

A number of authors report newborns who have been born with clinical and laboratory evidence of intoxication, when mothers have presented in labor in a drunken state or have been given alcohol intravenously to retard labor.

Alcohol withdrawal syndrome has also been reported in infants of chronically alcoholic women who were intoxicated at delivery. Withdrawal symptoms have included jitteriness, coarse tremors of the hands and feet, general restlessness, sleeplessness, excessive crying, and hyperirritability. Unlike infants with narcotic withdrawal, gastrointestinal signs such as vomiting or diarrhea have not been observed.

Growth abnormalities Initial growth studies of maternal alcoholism were retrospective. The examiners knew the mother's drinking history prior to assessment of the babies. Since that time a number of studies have been carried out in the United States and Europe. A consistent finding in these studies has been that children born to heavy-drinking women are generally smaller at birth.[14,18-20] In the Boston City Hospital study,[14] prematurity rose from 5% in the abstinent and 3% in the moderate groups to 17% in the heavy-drinking group. Women were interviewed at the first prenatal visit concerning alcohol intake, nutrition, smoking, caffeine, and the use of other psychoactive drugs. Alcohol intake was assessed using the scoring of Cahalan et al.[15] In this study, heavy drinking was defined as a consistent daily average intake of at least 45 ml of absolute alcohol plus the consumption of five or more drinks on one occasion. Most women were reinterviewed following delivery to assess the consistency of responses. Most women in this study did not meet all the minimal daily requirements prescribed by the Food and Nutrition Board of the National Academy of Science/National Research Council, but there were no differences in nutrition across the three drinking groups. Laboratory determinations of nutrients were not obtained in the study. In calculating all data, maternal age, parity, nutrition, smoking, and caffeine intake were controlled for.

It has been noted that the length of some of these children has been more affected than their weight. In addition, postnatal growth retardation has been documented in some cases in spite of adequate nutritional intake.

Growth hormone has been studied in a number of children with alcohol embryopathy. Results have shown a normal or slight hyper-response of growth hormone up to 150 ng/ml, with normal somatomedin activity in those blood samples with high growth hormone levels. It would appear that growth retardation in these cases does not result from deficiency in either growth hormone or somatomedin.

Root et al[21] have carried out studies of hypothalamic-pituitary function in 4 children born to the same alcoholic mother. Serum concentrations of growth hormone, insulin, follicle-stimulating hormone, luteinizing hormone, and parathyroid hormone were determined. Bone age was assessed by roentgenograms of the hands and wrists. All the biochemical and endocrine studies were normal. Bone ages were in advance of height ages in all 4 children studied. In this study 3 of the 4 children were underweight for height, implying that nutritional factors were contributing to short stature.

Congenital anomalies   One of the hallmarks of the effects of maternal alcoholism has been the increased frequency of congenital abnormalities found in the offspring of heavy-drinking women as compared with the general population. At the present time, the risk of an abnormal pregnancy outcome to women who drink heavily is still unknown.

Ouellette et al[22] found that the frequency of all abnormalities in the offspring of heavy drinkers increased twofold, as compared with abstainers and moderate drinkers. Thirty-two percent of infants born to heavy-drinking women had some form of congenital anomaly, as compared to 9% born to abstinent mothers and 14% to moderate drinkers. Both major and minor anomalies were more common. Minor anomalies were seen in 15% of infants born to heavy-drinking women, as compared to 5% and 12% of babies born to abstinent and moderate-drinking women, respectively. Major anomalies rose from 3% to 2% in the abstinent and moderate groups to17% in the heavy-drinking group. Multiple congenital anomalies occurred in 3% and 5% of the abstinent and moderate-drinking group, and rose to 20% among offspring born to heavy-drinking women. Sixty-seven percent of heavy-drinking women who significantly reduced their alcohol intake during pregnancy, or abstained altogether, had normal babies. These findings serve to re-emphasize the critical importance of identifying pregnant women at risk early in their pregnancies and providing them with appropriate counseling.

There is some evidence that the severity of abnormalities increases in offspring of each successive pregnancy in which the mother continues to drink heavily. It is important for physicians to be aware of this risk in order to initiate appropriate counseling.

Information on the possible role of moderate maternal drinking on pregnancy outcome is incomplete and contradictory. No nutritional data have been reported in any of the published clinical studies. Safe levels of alcohol intake during pregnancy, if any, have not yet been determined. No clinical information exists currently concerning any possible influence on the fetus of excessive paternal drinking prior to or at conception.

Animal Research

Results of heavy ethanol intake in animal research have been mixed and contradictory. Often insufficient information has been given to allow assessment of the adequacy of nutritional controls. Experimental designs have varied and probably account for the multiplicity of findings.

In growth studies the findings have generally been consistent with clinical reports. Fetuses and newborn animals born to pregnant females fed high doses of ethanol have weighed less than the control pups.

A number of recent studies have resulted in the production of fetal malformations that are strikingly similar to the congenital anomalies in humans. In the most elegant of these studies, Randall et al[23] fed an experimental group of mice a liquid diet with 25% of the total daily calories supplied by ethanol from gestation day 5 through gestation day 10. Isocaloric pair-fed controls were utilized. All anomalies were verified by at least two observers, one of whom was unaware of whether the fetus was part of the experimental or the control group.

A large number of skeletal and heart anomalies were observed in fetuses of alcohol-fed mothers. Limb anomalies included syndactyly, adactyly, and ectrodactyly of the forelimbs with occasional distortion of digits of the hind limbs. No limb anomalies were observed in control fetuses. Cardiovascular anomalies included abnormalities of both the major branches of the aorta and vena caval system, and intracardiac anomalies such as atresia of the mitral valves and interventricular septal defects. Urogenital anomalies were found in 8 experimental and 1 control fetus. Hydronephrosis and/or hydroureter of varying degrees, both bilateral and unilateral, were noted. Gastroschisis was noted in some fetuses. Head anomalies in the experimental group included 1 case of exencephaly and 2 of hydrocephalus. One case of anophthalmia and 3 cases of microphthalmia were noted.

Chernoff[24] also provided between 15% and 35% ethanol-derived calories to mice and found a dose-response effect and strain differences in susceptibility to alcohol. Study diet composition was controlled, but actual intake was not controlled.

Decreased fertility, increased prenatal and perinatal mortality, and increased fetal resorption have all been described in a variety of mammals whose mothers have been fed large doses of ethanol during pergnancy. Survival times of rats whose nursing mothers were fed ethanol has been found to be diminished.

Only one study has been published concerning the effect of moderate ethanol consumption during gestation in animals. Oisund et al[25] fed ethanol as 20% to 25% of total calories to rats for three to four weeks prior to, during, and also after pregnancy in some experiments. Isocaloric pair-fed controls were used. They found a statistically significant reduction in litter size after ethanol feeding, but no other statistically significant differences were found in body or organ weights between experimental and control rats. Two gross malformations were found among 321 ethanol-treated pups, whereas no malformations were found in 444 control pups. The authors concluded that moderate ethanol consumption by rat mothers did not have serious effects on their reproductive performance.

168

Discussion

Although it is clearly established that ethanol crosses the placenta and rapidly moves into the fetal circulation, tissues, and amniotic fluid, the means by which alterations in fetal growth and malformations occur are not well understood. A number of mechanisms can be postulated to explain the effects of heavy drinking during pregnancy on offspring. These effects may not be mutually exclusive but may prove to be additive.

Because alcohol crosses the placenta and is found in fetal tissues within 30 minutes of maternal ingestion, it in itself may be producing some harmful effects. Alcohol acts as a central nervous system depressant in postnatal life and it may exert direct effects on enzyme systems and/or protein synthesis, thus affecting growth and morphogenesis.

Rawat[26] has pointed out that proteins play an important role in the brain in intelligence, learning, and retention of memory. A decrease in protein synthesis during fetal life could result in growth retardation and affect central nervous system functioning in other ways. Rawat has demonstrated that continuous drinking of alcohol by pregnant rats leads to a marked decrease in the formation of proteins in the brain, liver, and heart.

Ethanol itself may be interfering with the normal development of neurotransmitters in the central nervous system. Studies have shown that maternal alcohol consumption results in decreases in brain dopamine, RNA, and DNA.

Metabolic breakdown products of alcohol may also contribute to the growth abnormalities and teratogenic effects seen clinically. Acetaldehyde is known to be a very toxic agent. It also crosses the placenta and may be producing harmful effects. Fetal enzymes that degrade ethanol are also increased by maternal alcohol ingestion and may play some role in the production of abnormalities. The microsomal ethanol-oxidizing system in the mouse fetus rises correspondingly with a rise in the maternal blood alcohol level. It is not yet known whether this enzymatic rise may be contributing to the production of malformations.

Hypoglycemia   Alcohol intake results in a fall in blood sugar and may produce ketoacidosis and significant hypoglycemia in some cases, particularly when ingested by children. The effects of hypoglycemia on the fetus are not well-defined. Infants of diabetic mothers have a greatly increased frequency of significant congenital anomalies. Although this is thought to be due in part to the effects of insulin, alterations in fetal blood sugar may play a role. It is possible that the intake of a large amount of alcohol at one time early in a mother's pregnancy may produce significant hypoglycemia in the fetus and result in the production of malformations. It is also possible that infrequent consumption of large amounts of alcohol may be more dangerous in this respect than more frequent consumption of small amounts of alcohol. There is no research confirmation of this hypothesis at this time.

Vitamin deficiencies   The effects on the fetus of maternal vitamin deficiency during pregnancy are not well understood. Chronic alcohol abuse is known to be associated with deficiencies in a number of vitamins and other nutrients. Thiamine, pyridoxine, and folic acid deficiencies have been studied extensively in adult alcoholics. Many of the hematologic, liver, and central nervous system changes seen in chronic alcoholics can be improved by the addition of these vitamins. Folic acid deficiency[27-29] in itself is known to produce spontaneous and repeated abortions, abruptions, premature births, and congenital malformations. A folic acid antagonist, aminopterin, has also been implicated in the production of congenital malformations.

Alcohol interferes with the intestinal absorption of folic acid. Studies have been carried out that show that when folic acid is given in the presence of alcohol, its uptake is decreased in the gut and adequate blood levels are not obtained. Folate-poor diets given with ethanol produce megaloblastic changes in the blood far more rapidly than when a folate-poor diet is given without ethanol. These findings suggest that ethanol administration may cause megaloblastic changes primarily when vitamin stores are decreased in the body and dietary intake is poor. Ethanol may act as a weak folate antagonist in these circumstances. It is possible that this antagonism to folate may be a contributing factor in the production of fetal malformations.

Blood levels of vitamins A, C, and folic acid have been measured in several mothers of clinically affected infants and have been found to be normal. Carefully controlled clinical and animal studies of isolated vitamin deficiencies on offspring have not yet been carried out.

Thiamine deficiency is difficult to produce by itself in the laboratory but is seen frequently with chronic alcoholism when nutritional intake has been poor. Central and peripheral nervous system changes, such as Wernicke's encephalopathy, Korsakoff's syndrome, and peripheral neuropathies are well described in adult alcoholics. Many of these can be reversed by thiamine treatment. Little is known about possible effects of maternal thiamine deficiency on the fetus. Careful studies need to be carried out to answer this question.

Amino acid deficiencies   Amino acid stores decrease naturally in women during pregnancy. Chronic alcohol intake prior to and during pregnancy may accentuate these deficiencies to a point where these vital building blocks of protein may become less available to the fetus. Zamenhof et al[30] have shown that separate omission of some single amino acids in pregnant rats resulted in decreased body and brain weights and decreased levels of cerebral DNA in their offspring. Further studies also need to be carried out in this field.

Trace metal deficiencies   Alcohol abuse has been shown to lower the quantity of trace metals in the body. Zinc and magnesium deficiencies have been documented in alcoholics. These trace metals are known to be important factors in producing memory loss in adult alcoholics due to their function in the hippocampus. Single deficiencies in these trace metals have been shown to produce congenital malformations in humans and laboratory mammals that are strikingly similar to those seen in offspring of alcoholic women. It is possible that chronic alcohol abuse may be producing its embryotoxic effects in part via deficiencies in these trace metals. Studies of the effects of these metals are currently in progress.

Malnutrition   Chronic alcohol abuse is very often associated with malnutrition, although some nutrients are present in alcoholic beverages. In most clinical studies the possible contributory effects of maternal malnutrition have not been positively excluded. In addition, many experimental studies carried out thus far have not controlled sufficiently for nutritional effects. Isocaloric pair-fed controls have not always been utilized. In some cases, no mention of any nutritional controls has been made. This renders conclusions drawn from these studies suspect until well-controlled studies have reproduced their effects.

Although nutritional influences are still not fully understood in the production of the fetal alcohol syndrome, there are a number of differences seen clinically in the offspring of chronically malnourished mothers that make it likely that malnutrition alone is not accounting for all the abnormalities seen. Smith[31] studied the effects of acute, self-limited, severe malnutrition on the outcome of pregnancy in several hundred women in Rotterdam, whose previous dietary intake had been adequate but who experienced severe nutritional deprivation for a nine-month period during World War II. This classic work demonstrated an increase in sterility, prematurity, small infants, and infant mortality, but malformed infants accounted for only 0.5% of the deliveries. Subsequent follow-up of this study[32] has shown that there is no difference in the outcome of these pregnancies 20 years later as compared to infants born in other parts of Holland during the same period.

More recent work in Latin America carried out by Cravioto et al[33] has demonstrated that diminished stature, head size, and intellectual accomplishments are seen in children of chronically malnourished mothers, but malformations were not noted to be increased in this group. Winick and Rosso[34] have demonstrated that both cerebral RNA and DNA are decreased in such children. Critical risk periods have been identified. Stoch and Smythe[35] have found in their South African studies that malnutrition in fetal and postnatal life has produced impaired body growth, particularly body weight, to a greater extent than body length. Cerebral growth tends to be spared. By contrast, infants of heavy-drinking women described thus far have shown a greater effect on head circumference and body length than on body weight. This discrepancy has been found to persist postnatally even when the diet has been shown to be adequate. In addition, some mothers of infants afflicted with growth and congenital malformations have been followed prenatally, and clinically significant malnutrition has not been demonstrated.

A number of animal studies,[36,37] well-controlled for nutrition, have demonstrated abnormalities in offspring of alcohol-fed mammals that are strikingly similar to those seen clinically in children of alcoholic women. These data are more convincing in ruling out malnutrition alone as a causative factor in the production of fetal abnormalities. Malnutrition, or relative malnutrition, may play an additive role in the production of growth' abnormalities, but it appears likely that it cannot be cited as the sole cause of the full range of abnormalities thus far described.

Other possible factors   Infants of drug-addicted mothers have been found to show withdrawal symptoms in the newborn period. Seizures have occurred in some of these babies, particularly those born to women maintained on methadone programs. Maternal malnutrition has also been noted in a number of these cases. Although prematurity and neonatal mortality rates are increased in this group, growth abnormalities and an increase in congenital anomalies have never been substantiated. In the study by Ouellette et al[22] maternal drug abuse during pregnancy was seen in less than 5% of pregnancies in the study group at Boston City Hospital, and the outcome of these pregnancies was not significantly different from those in which drug abuse was not present. Mothers with heavy alcohol intake admitted to a greater amount of previous drug use than abstainers or moderate drinkers. However, it appears unlikely that drug abuse plays any significant role in the production of the abnormalities seen with maternal alcohol abuse.

Smoking during pregnancy is associated with intrauterine growth retardation, increased frequency of premature and small-for-gestational-age infants, and an increase in infant mortality. In general, heavy drinkers tend to be heavy smokers. Clinical studies have not always been able to separate the effects of smoking from the effects of alcohol. Current evidence, however, shows that smoking itself does not cause congenital malformations. Additional studies need to be carried out to separate the possible contributing effects of heavy smoking from heavy drinking in the production of fetal abnormalities.

Little is known about any possible contributing effects of caffeine to the production of alcohol embryopathy. Caffeine intake is usually increased in those who smoke and drink heavily.

Prevention

At the present time, there is no known way to reverse or reduce the

172

effects of alcohol embryopathy once they have occurred. Supportive therapy, stimulation, and special education are the primary treatment modes.

It must be stressed that this is a totally preventable cause of growth abnormalities, congenital malformations, and mental retardation. Extensive efforts should be made to educate young women concerning the possible hazards of excessive alcohol ingestion prior to and during pregnancy. Junior-high and high schools are proving to be excellent sites for early education about the risks of alcohol abuse during pregnancy. Family planning and prenatal clinics are also important locations for educational programs and places where women with alcohol problems should be identified and referred for counseling.

The specific risk of producing an abnormal infant to a pregnant mother who is drinking large amounts of alcohol is currently unknown. Safe levels of alcohol ingestion during pregnancy, if any, have not been determined. Some evidence exists that decreasing or omitting alcohol use after pregnancy has begun increases the likelihood of having a normal child.

Women should be questioned about their drinking habits as well as their general nutrition, smoking, and other pertinent health information at the time of the first prenatal visit. Answers that indicate that a drinking problem may be present should be carefully noted and the woman referred to an appropriate treatment center for subsequent counseling. Rosett et al[38] found that pregnancy is an ideal time to intervene with a woman with a drinking problem. Women are motivated at this time to do what is best for their infant and regularly seek care from health care deliverers. Only if these health care deliverers are alert to the existence of the problem, identify young women at risk for alcohol problems, and educate and counsel them, can this significant cause of pediatric morbidity be diminished and ultimately abolished.

REFERENCES

1. Haggard HW, Jellinek EM: *Alcohol Explored*. Garden City, NY, Doubleday-Doran & Company, 1942.

2. Christiaens, L, Mizon JP, Delmarle G: On the descendants of alcoholics. *Ann Pediatr* 36:37–42, 1960.

3. Sandberg DH: Drugs in pregnancy: their effects on the fetus and newborn. *Calif Med* 94:287–291, 1961.

4. Shaeffer O: Alcohol withdrawal syndrome in a newborn infant of a Yukon Indian mother. *Can Med Assoc J* 87:1333–1334, 1962.

5. Lemoine P, Harousseau H, Borteyru JP, et al: Les enfants de parents alcooliques: anomalies observées. *Ouest-Medical* 25:476–481, 1968.

6. Ulleland C: The offspring of alcoholic mothers. *Ann NY Acad Sci* 197:167–168, 1972.

7. Ulleland C, Wennberg RP, Igo RP, et al: The offspring of alcoholic mothers (abs no. 152). *Pediatr Res* 4:474, 1970.

8. Jones KL, Smith DW: Recognition of the fetal alcohol syndrome in early infancy. *Lancet* 2:999–1001, 1973.

9. Jones KL, Smith DW: Offspring of chronic alcoholic women. Letter. *Lancet* 2:349, 1974.

10. Jones KL, Smith DW, Streissguth AP, et al: Outcome in offspring of chronic alcoholic women. *Lancet* 1:1076–1078, 1974.

11. Jones KL, Smith DW, Ulleland C, et al: Pattern of malformation in offspring of chronic alcoholic mothers. *Lancet* 1:1267, 1973.

12. Linbeck VL: The woman alcoholic. A review of the literature. *Int J Addict* 7:567–580, 1972.

13. National Institute on Alcohol and Alcoholism: *Second Report to US Congress.* Washington, DC, US Department of Health, Education and Welfare, 1974, p 5.

14. Ouellette EM, Rosett HL: A pilot prospective study of the fetal alcohol syndrome at the Boston City Hospital. Part II. The infants. *Ann NY Acad Sci* 273:123–129, 1976.

15. Cahalan D, Crisin I, Crossley H: *American Drinking Practices: A National Study of Drinking Behavior and Attitudes.* New Brunswick, NJ, Rutgers University Press, 1969.

16. Little RE, Streissguth AP: Moderate alcohol use during pregnancy and decreased infant birth weight. *Am J Public Health* 67:1154–1157, 1977.

17. Shaw S, Leiber CS: Plasma amino acids, and albumin synthesis. III. Effects of ethanol, acetaldehyde, and 4-methylpurazole. *Gastroenterology* 74:677–682, 1978.

18. Hanson JW, Streissguth AP, Smith DW: The effects of moderate alcohol consumption during pregnancy on fetal growth and morphogenesis. *J Pediatr* 92:457–460, 1978.

19. Kaminski M, Rumeau-Rouquette C, Schwartz D: Consumption of alcohol among pregnant women and outcome of the pregnancy. *Rev Epidemiol Sante Publique* 24:27–40, 1976.

20. Ouellette EM, Rosett HL: The effect of maternal alcohol ingestion during pregnancy on offspring, in Moghissi KS, Evans TN (eds): *Nutrition and Human Reproduction: Biochemical and Clinical Aspects.* New York, Harper & Row Publishers Inc, 1976, pp 107–120.

21. Root AW, Reiter EO, Andriola M, et al: Hypothalamic pituitary function in the fetal alcohol syndrome. *J Pediatr* 87:585–588, 1975.

22. Ouellette EM, Rosett HL, Rosman NP, et al: Adverse effects in offspring of maternal alcohol abuse during pregnancy. *N Engl J Med* 297:528–530, 1977.

23. Randall CL, Taylor J, Walker DW: Ethanol-induced malformations in mice. *Alcoholism* 1:219–223, 1977.

24. Chernoff GF: The fetal alcohol syndrome in mice: an animal model. *Teratology* 15:223–229, 1977.

25. Oisund JF, Fjorden AE, Morland J: Is moderate ethanol consumption teratogenic for the rat? *Acta Pharmacol Toxicol* 43:145–155, 1978.

26. Rawat AK: Ribosomal protein synthesis in the fetal and neonatal rat brain as influenced by maternal ethanol consumption. *Res Commun Chem Pathol Pharmacol* 12:723–732, 1975.

27. Folacin deficiency in alcoholism. *Nutr Rev* 22:8, 1964.

28. Folacin deficiency in pregnancy. *Nutr Rev* 25:166–168, 1967.

29. Folic acid and pregnancy. *Nutr Rev* 26:5–8, 1968.

174

30. Zamenhof S, Van Marshens E, Margolis FL: DNA (cell number) and protein in neonatal brain: alteration by maternal dietary protein restriction. *Science* 160:322-323, 1968.

31. Smith CJ: Effects of maternal undernutrition upon the newborn infant in Holland (1944-1945). *J Pediatr* 30:229, 1947.

32. Streissguth AP: Fetal alcohol syndrome: an epidemiologic perspective. *Am J Epidemiol* 107:467-478, 1978.

33. Cravioto J, Delicardie ER, Birch HC: Nutrition, growth and neurointegrative development: an experimental and ecologic study. *Pediatrics* 38(suppl 2):319, 1966.

34. Winick M, Rosso P: The effect of severe early malnutrition on cellular growth of human brain. *Pediatr Res* 3:181, 1969.

35. Stoch MB, Smythe PM: Does undernutrition during infancy inhibit brain growth and subsequent intellectual development. *Arch Dis Child* 38:546, 1963.

36. Randall CL, Taylor WJ: Prenatal ethanol exposure in mice: teratogenetic effects. *Teratology* (In press).

37. Rawat AK: Developmental changes in the brain levels of neurotransmitters as influenced by maternal ethanol consumption in the rat. *Neurochemistry* 28:1175-1182, 1977.

38. Rosett HL, Ouellette EM, Weiner L, et al: Therapy of heavy drinking during pregnancy. *Obstet Gynecol* 51:41-46, 1978.

15 Dietary Fiber and Cancer

David Kritchevsky, PhD
Jon A. Story, PhD

There is considerable current interest in the role of dietary fiber in the etiology of a number of diseases prevalent in the Western world. Prominent among those disease states whose prevalence is correlated with diets deficient in fiber is cancer of the large bowel. The high level of interest in the fiber hypothesis is due, in large part, to the epidemiologic observations of Burkitt and his colleagues[1-3] who perceived that one factor common among diseases of the large bowel was a diet low in fiber. Drasar and Irving,[4] on the other hand, correlated incidence of breast and colon cancer with a number of environmental factors and found a high positive correlation with total fat and animal protein, but practically none with dietary fiber (Table 15-1).

These apparently mutually exclusive observations may be explained when we consider that populations that ingest a diet high in animal products generally eat little fiber. Leveille[5] has recently reviewed the correlations between diet and incidence of cancer in Connecticut men, a group that exhibits one of the world's highest rates of colon cancer. Leveille reviewed the annual consumption of beef, meat, poultry, fish, cereals, and potatoes in

176

Table 15-1
**Correlation Between Dietary Components
and Incidence of Colon Cancer**

Component	Correlation Coefficient
Fat	
Total	0.81
Animal	0.84
Protein	
Total	0.70
Animal	0.87
Refined sugar	0.32
Fiber and complex carbohydrates	
Total	0.02
Potatoes and starches	− 0.07
Nuts	0.07
Fruit	0.22
Cereals	− 0.32

Reprinted from Drasar and Irving[4] with permission.

this population (Table 15-2). Between 1935 and 1965 the incidence of
colon cancer among Connecticut males had risen by 35%; consumption of
beef and other meats had risen by 55% and 36%, respectively, whereas consumption of cereals had decreased by 30% and potatoes by 26%.

Table 15-2
**Incidence of Cancer of the Large Intestine in Connecticut
Men* as Related to US Dietary Changes**

Period	Cancer/10⁵†	Annual Per Capita Consumption (lb)			
		Beef	MPF‡	Cereal	Potatoes
1935–38	19.7	44	148	205	149
1939–42	21.2	46	165	200	140
1943–46	23.9	45	182	198	142
1947–49	25.9	51	176	170	121
1950–53	27.2	51	179	163	112
1954–57	28.9	65	192	151	111
1958–61	30.0	63	194	148	109
1962–65	30.4	68	201	144	110

After Leveille.[5] Reprinted with permission
*Age-adjusted.
†Incidence of cancer per 100,000 population.
‡Meat, poultry, and fish.

Statistical analysis showed a high positive correlation with ingestion of beef and meat, poultry, and fish, and an even higher negative correlation with consumption of cereals and potatoes (Table 15-3). However, all of the dietary data reveal association, not causality, and must be interpreted with caution.

Table 15-3
Correlation Between Cancer of the Large Intestine in Connecticut Men and Consumption of Certain Foodstuffs

Consumption of	Correlation Coefficient
Beef	+ 0.905
Meat, poultry, and fish	+ 0.941
Cereals	− 0.974
Potatoes	− 0.968

After Leveille.[5] Reprinted with permission.

Assuming that a diet high in fiber gives protection against colon cancer, what is the mechanism of fiber's action? Fiber in the diet shortens intestinal transit time of food and, hence, shortens residence time of potential carcinogens.[6] Many types of fiber exhibit water-holding properties and, in this way, increase fecal bulk and peristaltic action.[7] It has also been suggested that the intestinal flora interact with fiber to produce volatile fatty acids that exert a laxative effect.[7]

Another mechanism of action involves the indirect effects of fiber on bile acid metabolism. In 1933, Wieland and Dane[8] were able, in the laboratory, to convert deoxycholic acid to methylcholanthrene, a very potent carcinogen. Deoxycholic acid itself has been found to be carcinogenic when applied to mouse skin.[9] These are two instances in which a bile acid is related in some fashion to carcinogenesis. Intestinal conversions of cholesterol and natural bile salts to metabolic products often found in the feces are accomplished by various intestinal microflora. Association of certain fecal steroid products with incidence of cancer and with levels of various types of bacteria yields data for further speculation.

Reddy et al[10] have presented data on the spectrum of fecal steroids found in patients with colon cancer (Table 15-4). They showed that patients with colon cancer excreted 185% more neutral steroids and 68% more bile acids than did controls. Further examination of the data shows that the ratio of cholesterol to coprostanol is increased in the cancer patients and the ratio of primary (biosynthesized) to secondary (metabolic products) bile acids is reduced. Coprostanol and the secondary bile acids are products of bacterial action. The ratio of undetermined fecal bile acids to total bile acids in controls (33.6%) and colon cancer patients (36.8%) is practically the same. Figure 15-1 depicts the primary and secondary bile acids.

Figure 15-2 shows the conversion of cholesterol to coprostanol. In

178

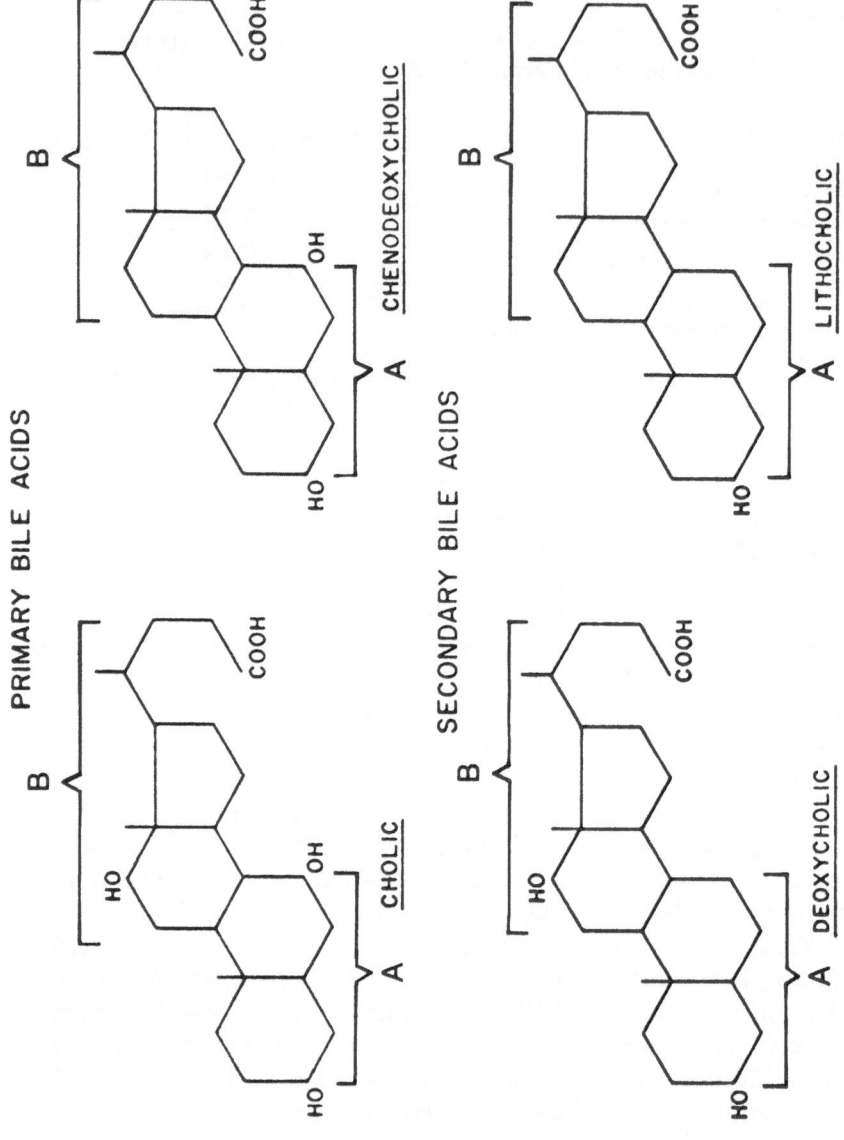

Figure 15-1 Primary and secondary bile acids.

Table 15-4
Fecal Steroids (mg/g) in Patients with Colon Cancer

	Patients (n = 12)	Patients (n = 15)
Neutral		
Cholesterol (A)	13.8	3.8
Coprostanol (B)	23.0	12.6
A/B	0.60	0.30
Acidic		
Cholic acid	0.6	0.9
Chenodeoxycholic acid	0.4	0.2
Deoxycholic acid	7.2	4.2
Lithocholic acid	5.7	3.4
Other	8.1	4.4
P/S*	0.08	0.14

After Reddy et al.[10] Reprinted with permission.
*Primary (cholic and chenodeoxycholic)/Secondary (deoxycholic and lithocholic) bile acids.

Figure 15-3, we see the metabolic steps that convert a bile salt to a free bile acid (via a hydrolase) and then convert the bile acid, cholic acid in this case, to ketone derivative by the action of a 7-dehydrogenase or to a secondary bile acid (deoxycholic) via a 7-dehydroxylase. These metabolic capabilities are all found in intestinal bacteria.

Hill[11] has reviewed the evidence that supports the theory that bile salts may be converted to carcinogenic hydrocarbons by bacterial action. The major reactions (Figure 15-3) have been demonstrated in vivo. Other reactions that would aromatize rings A and B (see Figure 15-1) have been carried out in vitro using human intestinal bacteria.

Hill[11] has also reported which particular strains of bacteria exhibit the metabolic actions shown in Figure 15-3. Thus, no *Escherichia coli* strains have hydrolase or dehydroxylase activity, but 78% show 7α-dehydrogenase activity. *Streptococcus salivarius, S. viridans,* and *Lactobacillus* species exhibit none of the enzymic activities, whereas among *S. faecalis* strains, 93% contain a hydrolase, 11% a dehydroxylase, and 81% have a 7α-dehydrogenase. Among strains of *Bacteroides fragilis,* 82% contain a hydrolase, 44% a dehydroxylase, and 79% a 7α-dehydrogenase (Table 15-5).

Hill argues that dietary fiber does not influence the excretion of steroids in man and summarizes data from several experiments (Table 15-6) that show that addition of varying amounts of bran to the diet of a number of subjects actually resulted in a reduction of fecal steroid output.

Nigro et al[12] examined the distribution of intestinal tumors experimentally induced with azoxymethane in rats fed a normal diet or one containing 2% of a bile salt-binding resin, cholestyramine. More tumors were

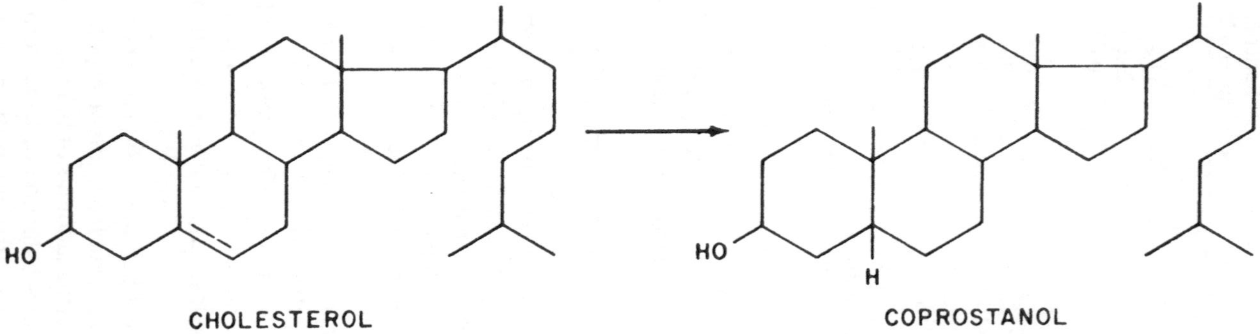

180

Figure 15-2 The conversion of cholesterol to coprostanol.

Table 15-5
Proportion of Strains of Gut Bacteria with Ability
to Metabolize Bile Acids and Bile Salts

Organism	No. per g of feces	Percentage with		
		Hydrolase	Dehydroxy- lase	7α-dehydro- genase
E coli	10^8	0	1	78
S faecalis	10^6	93	11	81
S salivarius	10^7	0	0	0
S viridans	10^7	0	0	0
Lactobacillus species	10^7	0	0	0
Bacteroides fragilis	10^{11}	82	44	79
Bifidobacterium species	10^{11}	74	40	56
Clostridium species	10^6	94	34	87
Veillonella species	10^4	50	4	50

After Hill.[11] Reprinted with permission.

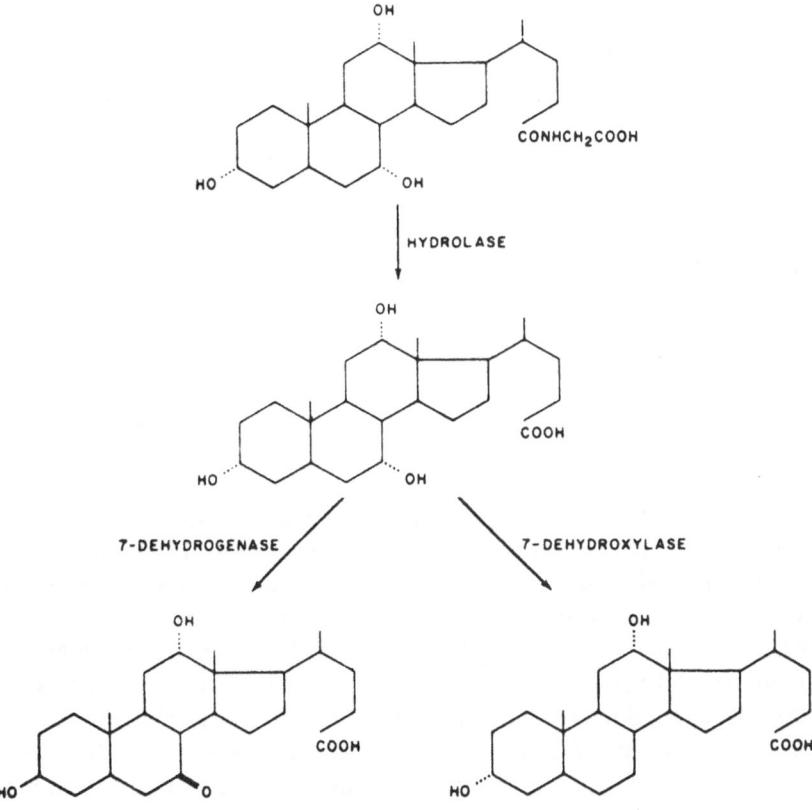

Figure 15-3   The metabolic steps in the conversion of bile salts to free bile acids (via a hydrolase).

Table 15-6
Effect of Fiber Intake on Fecal Steroids

Fiber (g/day)	No. Subjects	Weeks	% Control Value Neutral	% Control Value Acidic
Bran (16)	8	3	...	61
Bran (39)	4	4	63	63
Bran (100)	4	3	56	57
Bagasse (10.5)	10	12	61	100

After Hill.[11] Reprinted with permission.

observed on the cholestyramine-containing diet (Table 15-7). One explanation of this finding would be that bile acids or bile salts, even when bound, can act as cocarcinogens. It would have to be demonstrated, however, whether bile salts become metabolically inert when bound to a resin. Hill's hypothesis is that the intestinal flora, whose spectrum and activity are determined by diet, play the dominant role in colon carcinogenesis and that dietary fiber is of little consequence.

Table 15-7
Distribution of Intestinal Tumors in Rats Treated with Azoxymethane

Site of Tumor	No. of Tumors Normal Diet (n = 10)	No. of Tumors 2% Cholestyramine Diet (n = 10)
Small bowel		
Proximal	36	38
Distal	5	25
Large bowel		
Proximal	20	35
Distal	9	38

From Nigro et al.[12] Reprinted with permission.

Burkitt[13] has summarized data on colon cancer incidence, gut bacteria, and fecal steroids in six populations (Table 15-8). In the three populations with a high incidence of cancer (United States, Scotland, and England) the ratio of bacteroides to streptococci is 1.7 to 1.9, the ratio of neutral to acidic steroids is under 2.0, the daily intake of fat is high, and the intake of fiber is low. In the three populations with a low cancer incidence (Japan, South India, and Uganda) the ratio of bacteroides to streptococci is between 1.2 and 1.3, and the ratio of neutral to acidic steroids ranges from 3 to 5. Their fiber intake was 2 to 3 times that of the more susceptible populations. In the study of Reddy et al[10] (see Table 15-4), the ratio of neutral to acidic steroids was 1.7 in the cancer patients and 1.3 in the controls.

Table 15-8
Cancer of the Colon and Rectum, Bacterial Flora, and Fecal Steroids

	Population					
	United States	Scotland	England	Japan	South India	Uganda
Incidence per 100,000	41.6	51.5	38.1	13.1	14.0	3.5
Bacteria (log 10/g feces)						
Bacteroides	9.8	9.8	9.8	9.4	9.2	8.2
Streptococci	5.9	5.3	5.8	8.1	7.3	7.0
Fecal steroids (mg/g)*						
Neutral (N)	10.7 (64)	10.1 (77)	10.8 (69)	4.5 (43)	1.5 (62)	1.8 (55)
Acid (A)	6.0 (46)	6.2 (49)	6.2 (51)	0.9 (13)	0.5 (21)	0.5 (33)
N/A	1.78	1.63	1.74	5.00	3.00	3.60

After Burkitt.[13] Reprinted with permission.
*% degraded in parentheses.

Hill et al[14] generated most of the data quoted by Burkitt.[13] They obtained a virtually straight-line relationship when plotting total fecal dihydroxycholanoic acids against the incidence of colon cancer in six different populations. The ratio of anaerobic to aerobic bacteria present in the feces averaged 2.4 (range 2.1 to 2.7) in the populations with high rates of colon cancer, and 1.0 (range 0.5 to 1.5) in those with low rates of colon cancer.

If we assume that bile acids possess cocarcinogenic properties, then their prolonged presence alone may be sufficient to enhance carcinogenesis. Although bile acids have been shown to be cocarcinogenic for experimentally induced tumors,[15] it remains to be proven in vivo whether the findings were due to their metabolic or surface-active properties. In the latter case, any surface-active agent would be cocarcinogenic.

If the structure of a bile acid or salt affects its role in tumorigenesis, then the extent to which it is chemically or physically bound and rendered inert may be an important factor in reducing its activity. Animal feeding studies have shown that each type of fiber has its characteristic effect on steroid excretion. Thus, alfalfa[16] can increase excretion of neutral steroids whereas pectin[17] increases excretion of bile acids.

We have shown[18,19] that individual bile acids and salts are bound to different extents by different binding agents. As Figure 15-4 shows, cellulose has a weak binding capacity and cholestyramine a strong one. Among the natural binding substances lignin exhibits the greatest binding capacity. The binding for each substrate is shown in Figure 15-5. We see that lignin binds considerably more cholic acid than does alfalfa; their affinity for chenodeoxycholic acid is similar. When studying any specific bile acids or salts, their affinity for a variety of agents should be established.

184

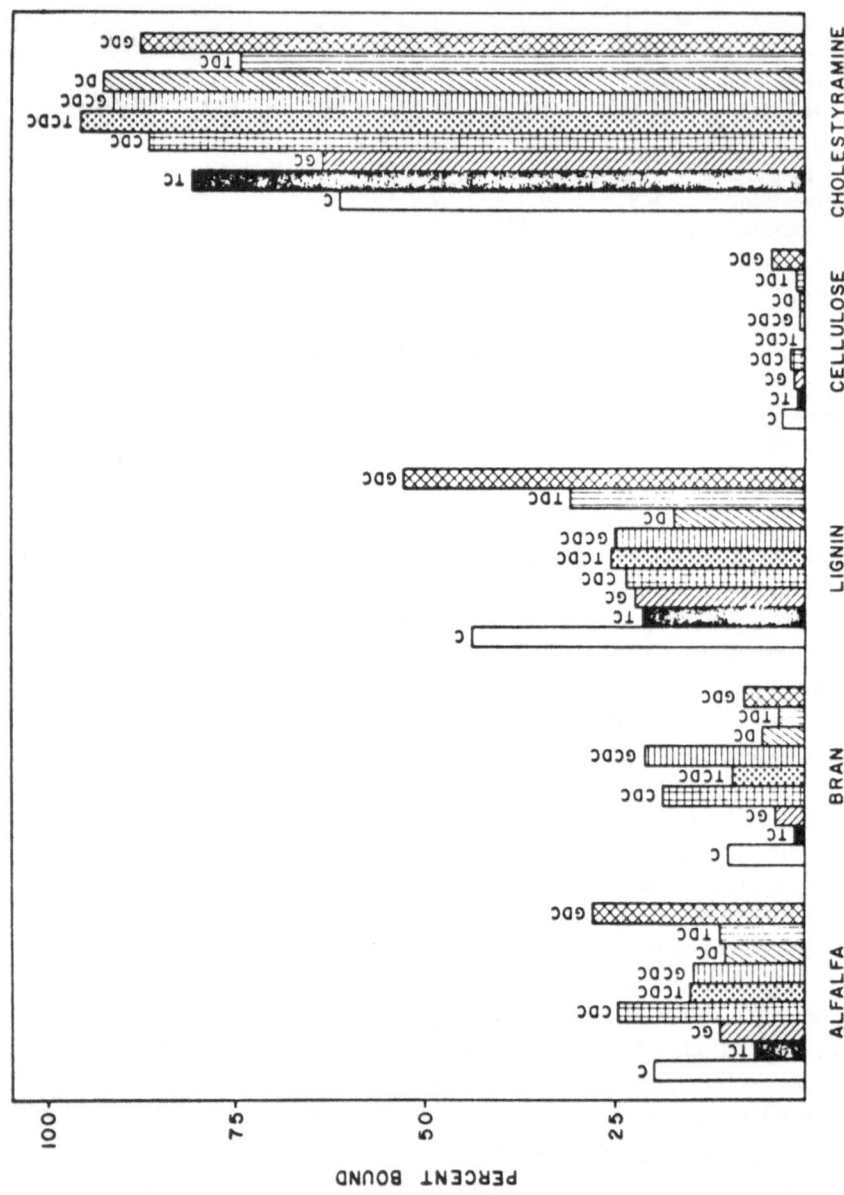

Figure 15-4 The effect of various binding agents on the bile acids and bile salts. C: cholic acid; TC: taurocholic acid; GC: glycocholic acid; CDC: chenodeoxycholic acid; TCDC: taurochenodeoxycholic acid; GCDC: glycochenodeoxycholic acid; DC: (carboxyl-¹⁴C)-deoxycholic acid; TDC: taurodeoxycholic acid; GDC: glycodeoxycholic acid.

185

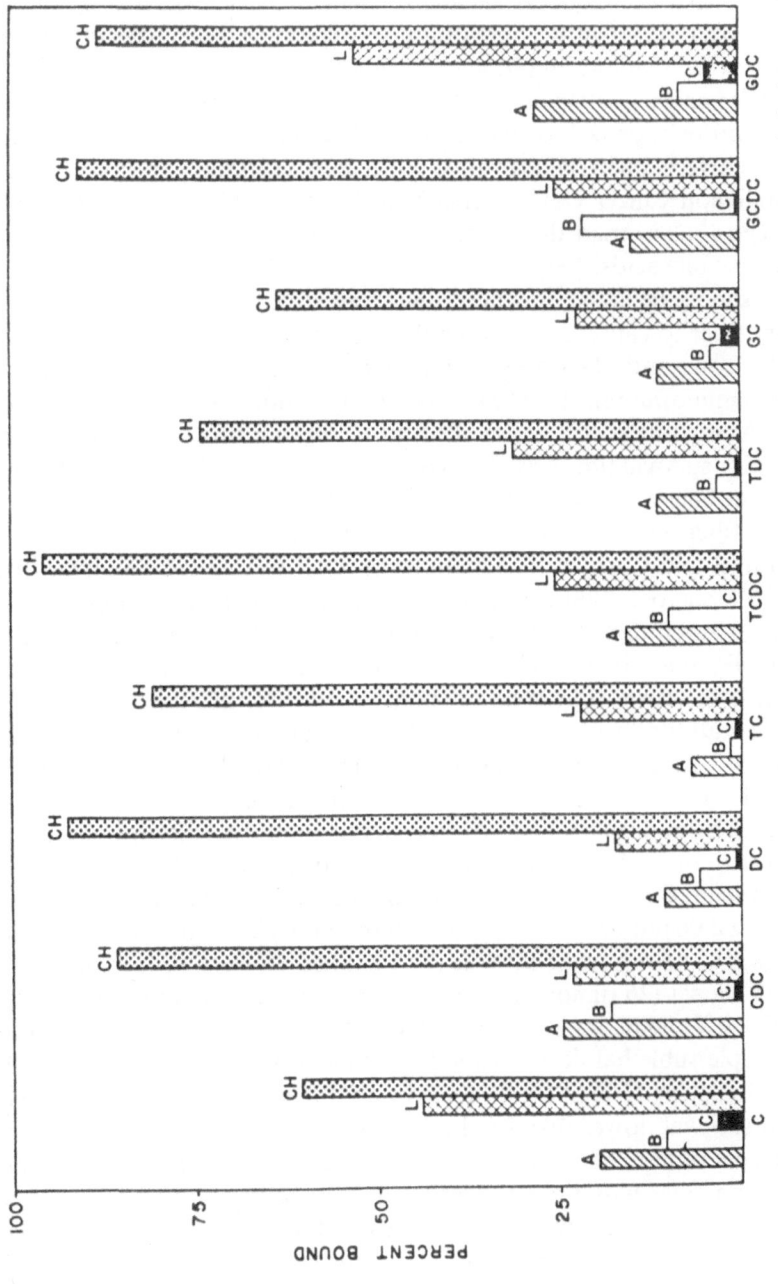

Figure 15-5 The percentage of bile acids and bile salts bound by alfalfa (A), bran (B), lignin (L), cellulose (C), and cholestyramine (CH). Abbreviation for bile acids and bile salts are the same as in Figure 15-4.

The production of colon cancer depends on the presence of a carcinogen and, probably, the length of time of exposure. If we accept the hypothesis that bile acids are potential precursors of carcinogens and we recognize that the required metabolic changes can be wrought by the intestinal bacteria, then it is important to determine which dietary factors influence bacterial proliferation. Examining the data summarized in Table 15-8, the incidence of colon cancer may be attributed to dietary fat, dietary animal protein, or lack of dietary fiber. Precisely how any of these components affects bacterial growth is under intense study.

If colon cancer can be related to dihydroxy bile acids,[14] it should be noted that in man dietary fiber can increase the level of primary to secondary bile acids.[20,21]

It should be noted, however, that there are a few experiments relating dietary fiber to cancers other than those of the large bowel.

Wilson and DeEds[22] compared the carcinogenic action of 2-acetylaminofluorene (AAF) in rats fed diets containing 3% or 6% crude fiber. At high levels of dietary AAF (0.125%) no difference in tumor incidence or survival time was observed, but when fed at the level of 0.062%, AAF was considerably less carcinogenic in the rats fed 6% fiber; rats fed the 3% fiber diet survived half as long as those fed the 6% fiber diet.

Engel and Copeland[23] administered AAF to rats fed a semipurified diet (70% sucrose, 18% casein, 6% lard, 5% salt mix, and 1% liver oil), a modified stock diet (61.5% whole wheat, 15% lard, 9.5% sucrose, 9% casein, 4% salt mix, and 1% cod liver oil), and a stock diet (61.5% whole wheat, 12% casein, 10% meat and bone scraps, 8% skim milk powder, 5% lard, 2% alfalfa leaf meal, 1% cod liver oil, and 0.5% iodized salt). The semipurified diet contained about 18% protein and 7% fat, the modified stock diet 15% protein and 18% fat, and the stock diet 27% protein and 9% fat. The major difference between the semipurified diet and the others was that most of the sucrose in the semipurified diet had been replaced by whole wheat. Over a large experimental series rats fed the semipurified diet exhibited 2.06 tumors per rat (97 tumors in 47 rats) in contrast to 1.5 tumors per rat (18 tumors in 12 rats) in the modified stock diet, and only 1.08 tumors per rat (26 tumors in 24 rats) in those animals fed the stock diet.

Ershoff and his co-workers[24] studied the influence of diet on the effects of multiple sublethal doses of total body x-ray irradiation in mice (Table 15-9). Replacing 15% of the dextrose by alfalfa leaf meal (diet 6) resulted in 53.3% survival, lower than on the basal diet, and the appearance of 1.75 tumors per mouse, higher than on the basal diet. This suggests that factors other than fiber may exert a major effect on survival and prevalence of tumors caused by x-ray irradiation. Still, if we use an arbitrary index (tumors per mouse $\times$ % survival) we find the values to be: 0.70, 1.17, 1.10, 0.47, 0.57, 0.93, and 0.23 for diets 1 through 7, respectively, the lowest value being observed in the group fed the stock diet.

Table 15-9
Influence of Diet on Tumors in X-ray Irradiated Mice
(Six Weekly Exposures to 200 rad)

Diet	Carbohydrate (%)	Fat (10%)*	Other (%)	T/m†	% Survival
1	Dextrose (59)	CSO	...	1.02	68.3
2	Dextrose (59)	Lard	...	2.33	50.0
3	Starch (59)	CSO	...	1.57	70.0
4	Dextrose (49)	CSO	Liver (10)	0.70	66.7
5	Dextrose (49)	CSO	Yeast (10)	0.87	50.0
6	Dextrose (44)	CSO	Alfalfa (15)	1.75	53.3
7	Stock	...	...	0.36	65.0

After Ershoff et al.[24]
*CSO = cottonseed oil.
†Tumors per mouse.

The question at the moment is of the chicken-egg variety, ie, which came first. In general, populations ingesting diets high in fiber do not eat a Western (or luxus) diet. More work is needed before we can safely ascribe enhancement or inhibition of carcinogenic potential to a specific dietary component.

REFERENCES

1. Burkitt DP: Some neglected leads to cancer causation. *JNCI* 47:913–919, 1971.
2. Burkitt DP: Epidemiology of cancer of the colon and rectum. *Cancer* 28:3–13, 1971.
3. Burkitt DP, Walker ARP, Painter NS: Dietary fiber and disease. *JAMA* 229:1068, 1974.
4. Drasar BS, Irving D: Environmental factors and cancer of the colon and breast. *Br J Cancer* 27:167, 1973.
5. Leveille GA: Issues in human nutrition and their probable impact on foods of animal origin. *J Anim Sci* 41:723–731, 1975.
6. Harvey RF, Pomare EW, Heaton KW: Effects of increased dietary fiber on intestinal transit. *Lancet* 1:1278–1280, 1973.
7. Cummings JH: Dietary fiber. *Gut* 14:69–81, 1973.
8. Wieland H, Dane E: The synthesis of methylcholanthrene. *Z Physiol Chem* 219:240–244, 1933.
9. Badger GM, Cook NW, Hewett CL, et al: Production of cancer by pure hydrocarbons. *Proc R Soc London [Biol]* 129:439–467, 1940.
10. Reddy BS, Mastromarino A, Wynder EL: Further leads on metabolic epidemiology of large bowel cancer. *Cancer Res* 35:3403–3406, 1975.
11. Hill MJ: Fecal steroids in the epidemiology of large bowel cancer, in Nair PP, Kritchevsky D (eds): *The Bile Acids,* vol 3. New York, Plenum Publishing Corporation, 1977, pp 169–200.

188

12. Nigro ND, Bhadrachari N, Chomchai C: A rat model for studying colonic cancer: effect of cholestyramine on induced tumors. *Dis Colon Rectum* 16:438, 1973.

13. Burkitt DP: Benign and malignant tumors of large bowel, in Burkitt DP, Trowell HC (eds): *Refined Carbohydrate Foods and Disease. Some Implications of Dietary Fiber.* London, Academic Press Inc, 1977, pp 117–133.

14. Hill MJ, Drasar BS, Aries VC, et al: Bacteria and the etiology of cancer of the large bowel. *Lancet* 1:95–100, 1971.

15. Reddy BS, Narisawa T, Maronpot R, et al: Animal models for the study of dietary factors and cancer of the large bowel. *Cancer Res* 35:3421–3426, 1975.

16. Kritchevsky D, Tepper SA, Story JA: Isocaloric, isogravic diets in rats. III. Effects of nonnutritive fiber (alfalfa or cellulose) on cholesterol metabolism. *Nutr Rep Int* 9:301, 1974.

17. Leveille GA, Sauberlich HE: Mechanism of the cholesterol-depressing effect of pectin in the cholesterol-fed rat. *J Nutr* 88:209–214, 1966.

18. Kritchevsky D, Story JA: Binding of bile salts *in vitro* by nonnutritive fiber. *J Nutr* 104:458–462, 1974.

19. Story JA, Kritchevsky D: Comparison of the binding of various bile acids and bile salts *in vitro* by several types of fiber. *J Nutr* 106:1292–1294, 1976.

20. Mathur KS, Khan MA, Sharma RD: Hypercholesterolaemic effects of Bengal gram: a long-term study in man. *Br Med J* 4:262–264, 1973.

21. Pomare EW, Heaton KW: Alteration of bile salt metabolism by dietary fiber (bran). *Br Med J* 4:262–264, 1973.

22. Wilson RH, DeEds F: Importance of diet in studies of chronic toxicity. *Arch Indust Hyg Occup Med* 1:73–80, 1950.

23. Engel RW, Copeland DH: Protective action of stock diets against the cancer-inducing action of 2-acetylaminofluorene in rats. *Cancer Res* 12:211, 1952.

24. Ershoff BH, Bajwa GS, Field JB, et al: Comparative effects of purified diets and a natural food stock ration on the tumor incidence of mice exposed to multiple sublethal doses of total-body x-irradiation. *Cancer Res* 29:780–788, 1969.

16 Nutrition and Chemotherapy — Drug-Nutrient Interactions Using Breast and Colon Carcinoma as Models

Richard J. Elkort, MD

Neoplastic disease grows within the confines of multicellular organisms. It comprises a new tissue which thrives at the expense of nearly every other normal tissue, with respect to space and true nutrition. In overall balance, the host withers, while the tumor flourishes. Furthermore, the host may suffer a wide variety of clinical effects from introduction of abnormal quantities of chemical substances from the tumor. These phenomena of space occupation, competition for critical nutrients, and tumor excretion underlie most of the diseases that cancers cause.[1]

The complexity of these problems is increased enormously when therapy is superimposed on the disease process. One can decrease these complexities to some extent by identifying and defining the major effects of some commonly used cancer chemotherapeutic drugs in relation to nutritional status.

Drug-nutrient interactions fall into two basic categories, direct and indirect. The indirect effects are brought about because many of the cancer chemotherapeutic drugs currently in use can impair absorption, increase excretion, or decrease utilization of various nutrients. Certain drugs can also lead to decreased nutrient intake because of attendant anorexia. The presence of malignancy itself, especially when it is systemic, is almost always associated with anorexia and most patients on chemotherapy will suffer some degree of gastrointestinal irritation manifested as nausea, vomiting, diarrhea, or stomatitis.[2] This results from the fact that rapidly dividing populations of cells are more sensitive to cancer chemotherapeutic agents than are more slowly dividing cells, and the gastrointestinal tract, the bone marrow, and the skin contain the most rapidly dividing cell populations in the body. For these reasons it is prudent to assume that all cancer patients under treatment will have some degree of malnutrition on the basis of anorexia, as well as greater or lesser degrees of malabsorption and excessive nutrient loss.

The direct drug effects are more subtle and less widely appreciated. A bewildering array of clinical findings involving virtually every organ system may be attributable to drug therapy, and the net result of all of these effects may be a significant change in the nutritional status of the patient. Physicians have only recently begun to consider the many ways in which drugs may influence the dietary intake of nutrients, their disposition in the body, and their rates of elimination. Conversely, the nutritional status of the patient may have a profound influence on the therapeutic efficacy of drugs and the likelihood of developing drug toxicity.

Newer techniques of biochemical evaluation of nutritional status are slowly becoming available to the medical profession, and at the present time it is possible to detect a wide range of disorders where drugs induce nutritional disorders. As a general rule, whenever a physician is considering the institution of cytotoxic therapy in a cancer patient in whom the impairment of nutrition can be reasonably assumed, appropriate nutrient supplementation should be considered; more especially, if the patient's diet has been inadequate or if he already has had disease-caused interference with nutrient absorption or utilization.

Model Tumor Systems

The tumor systems that have been selected for discussion involve those commonly encountered in the United States. Colorectal cancer is the most common malignancy in the United States for both sexes. Breast cancer is the most common malignancy seen in women today. Moreover, both of these tumors are treatable by a variety of modalities including surgery, radiotherapy, and chemotherapy, the latter producing a "cure" in some cases, especially when used in an adjuvant setting, and effective palliation in many other cases.

Two drug regimens have been selected for discussion, because of their widespread utilization and because they make use of drugs that have been available for study for many years. For breast cancer a widely studied program is the so-called CMF regimen using cyclophosphamide, methotrexate, and 5-fluorouracil. For colon cancer, 5-fluorouracil is commonly used in combination with a newer class of compounds, the nitrosoureas (carmustine [BCNU], lomustine [CCNU], and semustine [methyl CCNU]).

Cyclophosphamide belongs to the class of compounds known as alkylating agents; the nitrosoureas probably exert their effects in the same way on a molecular level. On the other hand, 5-fluorouracil and methotrexate are antimetabolites. In general, the remarks made relevant to these drugs will apply to most if not all of the drugs in the two classes of alkylating agents and antimetabolites. Taken together, these form the mainstay of cytotoxic cancer chemotherapy today.

Drug Characteristics

Methotrexate   Since their initial use in the treatment of acute lymphoblastic leukemia in 1948, the antifolate compounds and particularly methotrexate have become increasingly important in cancer chemotherapy. The antifolate compounds are protein inhibitors of dihydrofolate reductase, the enzyme that converts dihydrofolate to tetrahydrofolate and thus replenishes the intracellular pool of reduced folates required for thymidylate and purine synthesis, certain amino acid interconversions, and possibly the synthesis of neurotransmitters. The effects of the drug may be circumvented by giving leucovorin within 36 to 42 hours after administration of methotrexate. This supplies the metabolite blocked by the methotrexate and thereby neutralizes its biochemical effect.

Methotrexate is readily absorbed from the intestine and quickly bound to the dihydrofolate reductase enzyme. It displaces folate from the enzyme; this is followed by increased excretion of folate in the urine. Methotrexate does not inhibit folic acid absorption in man and the increased urinary excretion of the vitamin has been attributed to its displacement from binding sites on the reductase molecule and hence nonutilization. The induced folate deficiency can lead to megaloblastic anemia, hepatic fibrosis, and possibly cirrhosis.[3]

5-Fluorouracil is a fluorinated pyrimidine that is closely related in structure to uracil; it differs in the substitution of a fluorine atom for the hydrogen atom at carbon 5 of the uracil molecule. It inhibits tumor growth because of the special role of uracil as a precursor for nucleic acids. It is incorporated into RNA in place of uracil and subsequently interferes with the function of this RNA. It blocks the attachment of the methyl group to carbon 5 of uracil (an obligatory step in DNA precursor biosynthesis), and consequently it inhibits DNA synthesis. This activity is mediated by its inhibition of the enzyme thymidylate synthetase; it is felt that this action is mainly responsible for the tumor-inhibitory property of this compound. There are no clinically effective agents that will neutralize the therapeutic effect or toxicity of this compound.

Cyclophosphamide and lomustine (CCNU) These compounds will be considered together since they both act primarily as alkylating agents. An alkylating agent is a compound that directly or indirectly contributes an alkyl group, which becomes attached to some other compound, ion, or element. A biologic alkylating agent is one that can contribute an alkyl group under physiologic conditions of temperature and pH to a receptor entity that is a component of a biologic system.

Alkylation of molecules having low molecular weights usually produces little effect on the survival of cells, because the products may be excreted readily and the pools of small compounds replenished rapidly by biosynthesis. However, alkylation of macromolecules, particularly proteins and nucleic acids, probably has a more critical effect than the alkylation of small molecules, and it is likely that the products of such alkylations remain in the cells for longer periods of time. Polyfunctional alkylating agents, ie, those containing more than one binding site, are more effective than monofunctional alkylating agents since they cause cross-linking in double-stranded DNA molecules as well as cross-linking between protein and DNA or protein and RNA. All of these reactions are harmful to cell replication and survival.[3]

Most of the commonly used alkylating agents, including cyclophosphamide and two of the three currently used nitrosoureas, are absorbed from the gastrointestinal tract, but some of them, particularly the nitrogen mustards, are given intravenously because of their vesicant action.

The agents are widely distributed among the tissues with little or no preferential localization in neoplastic tissues. Several of the agents cross the blood-brain barrier only to a limited extent and are ineffective in killing neoplastic cells there. The nitrosoureas have relatively high lipid solubility, are essentially nonionized, and therefore are outstanding in crossing this barrier and have been effective in treating experimental neoplasms inoculated intracerebrally.

In one sense, the cytotoxic drugs can be effective only if they produce specific nutrient abnormalities. Problems arise because these defects are produced in normal cells as well as in the malignant cell population. When therapy produces a successful result it is because: 1) normal cells generally recover from the injurious effects of drug therapy more rapidly than do tumor cells; and 2) the relative proportion of tumor cells injured or destroyed is greater in relation to the total tumor cell population, than is the number of normal cells injured or destroyed in relation to the total number of normal cells in the target tissue or organ. As the relative numbers and/or drug resistance of tumor cells approaches that of normal cells, the effectiveness of cytotoxic therapy diminishes and its toxicity markedly increases.

In the case of critical nutrients, such as vitamins, additional therapeutic advantages may derive from special requirements of tumor metabolism that may apply in some cases. At least experimentally, deficiencies of folic acid, of pyridoxine, or of riboflavin have been found to result in significant inhibition of the growth of certain tumors beyond the effect of the vitamin deficiency per se.[4,5]

For the most effective use of cytotoxic chemotherapy, one must understand the metabolic requirements of normal and tumor tissue and manipulate the cellular microenvironment so as to favor the former and inhibit the latter.[6] Efforts to do this with nutrient modification alone have been disappointing. However, the use of controlled nutrition to increase the effectiveness of chemotherapeutic treatment programs has only recently begun to be explored and offers the best current hope for improving the results of such programs in the near future.

Current approaches are qualitative; they provide an excess of all nutrients in the hope that the organism will select what it needs from the substrates provided. In the ill patient these selective mechanisms may not operate effectively, and future progress in this area will depend on increasing the capability of the physician to provide quantitative nutrient support, providing those substrates that are helpful and withholding those that are not.

Drug-Nutrient Interactions

Combination chemotherapy programs usually are based on the use of cytotoxic compounds that have different mechanisms of action. For breast and colon cancer many of these programs utilize an alkylating agent and one or more antimetabolites, as has been described. Their indirect effects on nutrition are extremely variable in individual patients and have been summarized above. The direct effects include:

1. Folate deficiency.
2. Niacin deficiency.
3. Interference with protein biosynthesis (possible decrease in immune competence and host defenses against infection — atrophic changes in rapidly dividing tissues such as intestine, skin, and bone marrow).
4. Interference with glucose metabolism (hepatic effects).
5. Increased gluconeogenesis from endogenous protein.
6. Possible increased glycolysis and utilization of lipid reserves (ketosis).
7. Increased loss of fluid and electrolytes, particularly sodium chloride, due to vomiting and diarrhea.

194

8. Mineral deficiency, especially magnesium (tetany, muscle weakness, tremors) and zinc (impaired wound healing, hypogeusia).
9. Effects on the endocrine system, especially the pituitary-adrenal axis, with resultant variations (usually losses) in protein, calcium, and potassium.

Determination of how these variables can best be manipulated in order to enhance the patient's response to chemotherapy is the clinical nutritionist's further challenge.

REFERENCES

1. Roe DA: *Drug-Induced Nutritional Deficiencies.* Connecticut, Avi Publishing Company, 1976.
2. Holland JF: The diseases that cancer causes. *J Chronic Dis* 16:635–636, 1963.
3. Holland JF, Frei E: *Cancer Medicine.* Philadelphia, Lea & Febiger, 1973.
4. Rosen F, Mihich E, Nichol CA: Selective metabolic and chemotherapeutic effects of vitamin B_6 antimetabolites. *Vitam Horm* 22:609–641, 1964.
5. Morris HP, Robertson WV: Growth rate and number of spontaneous mammary carcinomas and riboflavin concentration of liver, muscle, and tumor of C3H mice as influenced by dietary riboflavin. *JNCI* 3:479–489, 1943.
6. Waterhouse C: How tumors affect host metabolism. *Ann NY Acad Sci* 230:86–93, 1974.

17 Diet and Diabetes Mellitus

Ronald A. Arky, MD

Diet is frequently said to be the principal therapeutic measure in the treatment of diabetes mellitus, yet a search of the literature reveals few substantial scientific data to corroborate the claim. What can diet therapy achieve in the treatment of the diabetic? Is there a "diabetic diet"? Does a diet high in carbohydrate content improve or aggravate diabetes? These questions are constantly posed to physicians and others involved in the therapy of diabetes. Yet for the most part, definitive answers are not available. Much of the approach to diet therapy of the diabetic has been based on tradition and misconceptions, and the quantity of recent investigative work relevant to nutrition and diabetes is very limited. The purpose of this review is to examine current concepts of the dietary approach to diabetes mellitus in the context of our understanding of the pathophysiology of the disorder. Admittedly, some personal biases will be evident, since strong investigative data are unavailable to confirm or deny traditional thinking.

What is Diabetes?

Dispute persists as to the level of hyperglycemia that is a sure indicator of diabetes.[1] Current concepts of the pathophysiology of this
heterogeneous syndrome recognize two basic lesions: one involves a
defect in the beta cells of the islets of Langerhans, and the second a
resistance to the effectiveness of insulin in peripheral tissues such as
muscle, liver, and adipose tissue (Figure 17-1). The complexity of the syndrome can be appreciated when it is recognized that both major defects may
be present in an absolute or relative degree, and that in some forms of
diabetes both defects may be involved. However, in clinical terms the first
lesion accounts for the majority of cases.

Mixed meals are absorbed after the various digestive processes have
broken down complex foodstuffs into their basic components. The anabolic processes that account for the storage of energy from absorbed
nutrients are modulated by insulin. Insulin secretion by the beta cells is
enhanced by "gut hormones" produced in the lower duodenum and upper
jejunum during the digestive process. Recent studies indicate that a
44–amino-acid peptide secreted by mucosal cells of the small intestine,
known as gastric inhibitory polypeptide, plays a major role in the release of
insulin.[2] In addition, absorbed nutrients such as glucose and amino acids
are also vital stimulators of insulin release.

Insulin enhances the uptake of nutrients by adipose tissue, muscle, and
other vital tissues. It effects this action by binding to specific protein recep-

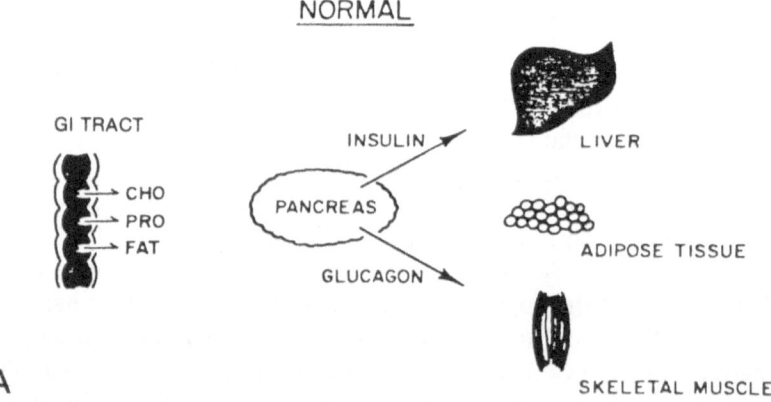

Figure 17-1 Pathophysiologic considerations in diabetes mellitus. **A** The postprandial pattern in normal individuals following mixed meals. Carbohydrates (CHO) and
amino acids derived from protein (PRO) stimulate the release of glucagon. Insulin
modulates the storage of carbohydrate as glycogen in liver and muscle, protein synthesis in muscle, and lipogenesis in adipose tissue. Glucagon will enhance hepatic
output of glucose if amino acid intake is excessive; however, the carbohydrate content of a mixed meal usually suppresses glucagon release.

tors on the membranes of these various tissues.[3] Other actions of insulin may be via second messengers or possibly by actions within the cell.[4] In the absence of insulin, anabolic processes come to a standstill and catabolic processes increase. Such a state exists in the insulin-requiring diabetic (ketone-prone or juvenile-type) who has not received insulin therapy. (The term juvenile-type diabetes is erroneous, as patients of all ages develop insulin-dependent diabetes; the term should be eliminated from the medical literature.)

The presence of insulin does not ensure a stable metabolism. For example, many obese individuals will have adequate quantities of circulating

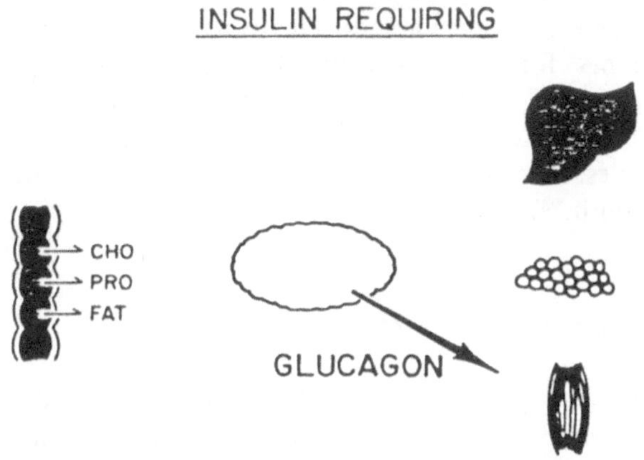

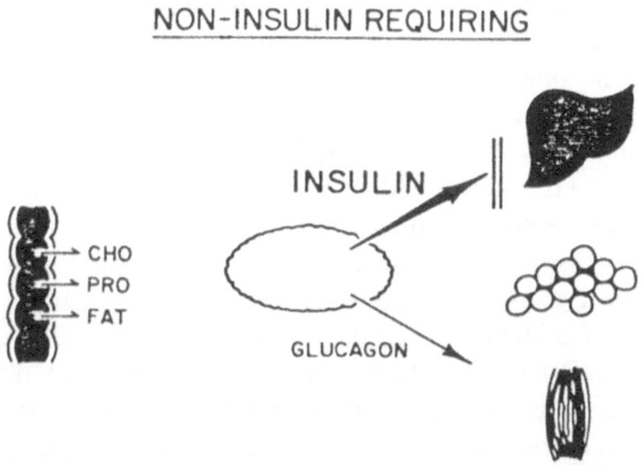

Figure 17-1B Pancreatic insulin output is zero after a mixed meal in insulin-requiring diabetics. Glucagon levels are relatively elevated in the face of hyperglycemia. If exogenous insulin is not administered, the postprandial milieu is catabolic, and Glycogenesis, protein synthesis, and lipogenesis are minimal. C Hyperinsulinemia characterizes the postprandial setting of many non-insulin-requiring diabetics, most of whom are obese. The actions of insulin are impeded. Weight reduction alleviates hyperinsulinism and the impedance to insulin's actions disappears.

insulin, yet demonstrate glucose intolerance. Several investigators have documented that the obese state is characterized by a reduced number of insulin receptors in the membranes of adipocytes, muscle, hepatocytes, and monocytes, and attribute the resistance to insulin's action in obese subjects in part to this defect. Other disease states characterized by insulin resistance may reflect alterations in the receptors or variations in the affinity of insulin for these receptors.[5]

In summary, diabetes is a complex heterogeneous syndrome that arises from two major pathologic defects: the first, a defective beta cell; the second, a resistance on the part of peripheral tissue to insulin. In clinical terms, the first lesion accounts for the majority of cases of insulin-dependent or ketone-prone diabetes. The second, or "peripheral resistance" lesion, accounts for the majority of cases of adult-onset diabetes (non–insulin-dependent, ketone-resistant). (The term adult-onset also warrants modification. Ketone-resistant, non–insulin-dependent diabetes may appear in adolescence and has been called by Fajans et al "maturity-onset diabetes of youth."[6])

General Principles of Dietary Therapy

Since the earliest descriptions of diabetes mellitus in the *Papyrus Ebers,* the major concern in the formulation of a diet for the treatment of the diabetic has centered about the relative amounts of the carbohydrate and fat content of such a diet. A chronologic summary of this debate is outlined in Table 17-1. Present thoughts are that this entire controversy is superfluous. The single most important objective in the dietary treatment of the diabetic is the control of total caloric intake.[7] Patients should be encouraged to ingest foods that are nutritionally adequate and sufficient in calories to achieve or maintain ideal body weight. Caloric intake should be adjusted so that the obese individual loses weight and so that youngsters and pregnant women with diabetes demonstrate normal growth and development. The diabetic diet should be designed to minimize glucosuria and the symptoms of diabetes. Since persistent and prolonged hyperglycemia has been associated with several of the complications of diabetes, diet therapy as well as the other therapeutic modalities should be aimed at preventing and/or delaying the development of these various complications.[8] When, however, a complication arises, such as that involving the kidneys, the diabetic diet must be modified to consider the diabetes as well as the associated problems. In addition to ensuring adequate carbohydrate, protein, and fat, the diet should have adequate amounts of minerals and vitamins. Diet therapy, just as therapy with hypoglycemic agents, must be integrated in the treatment plan with an activity schedule that emphasizes exercise and other means of expending energy.

Table 17-1
High Carbohydrate vs High Fat Diets for Diabetics

Advocates of High Carbohydrate-Low Fat Diets	
Papyrus Ebers	1500 BC
Aretaeus of Cappadocia	900 AD
Willis	1675
Protty	1857
Donkin	1869
Von During	1870
Dujarden-Beaumetz	1889
Mosse	1898
von Noorden	1902
Geyelin	1923
Adlersberg and Proges	1926
Sweeney	1927
Rabinowich	1931
Himsworth	1935
Kempner	1940
Van Eck	1961
Stone and Connors	1963
Ernest	1965
Brunzell	1971
Advocates of Higher Fat-Lower Carbohydrate Intake	
Rollo	1797
Pile	1860
Bouchardat	1872
Naunyn	1906
F.M. Allen	1912

From Wood and Bierman.[9] Reproduced with permission of *Nutrition Today* magazine, P.O. Box 1829, Annapolis, Maryland 21404, © May/June, 1972.

Rules for Diet Therapy

Most successful dietary programs for diabetics use a team approach.[10] All members of the team (physician, dietitian, nurse) must appreciate the importance of diet therapy and present a unified approach to the patient. The physician and dietitian should formulate a diet prescription that recognizes 1) the caloric needs of the patient; 2) the social, ethnic, and economic factors that control the patient's dietary habits; and 3) the patient's and/or his family's ability to comprehend the need for an altered or modified diet. In communities or settings where a team approach is impossible to develop, the physician must assume prime responsibility and make every effort to provide extensive and continuous diet counseling. In all instances, physicians should make every effort to locate a dietitian to assist the patient. (Local dietetic associations and regional affiliates of the American Diabetes Association are making efforts to establish referral services for diet counseling. Physicians unfamiliar with such services should address inquiries to their local American Diabetes Association affiliate.)

Before dietary instruction is possible, the dietary counselor (physician, dietitian, or nurse) must assess the ability of the patient to comprehend some of the basic principles of diet management. While the "exchange method" has been used in one form or another for the past 27 years and has recently been modified,[11] there are several other methods that can be approached and molded to the patient's and/or his family's ability to comprehend. Single encounters between the diet counselor and the patient are useless; altering an individual's life-long habits are not feasible in a single encounter. Just as a physician treating the diabetic reviews on each visit foot care and other basic principles, so should attention be given to the diet and the patient's compliance with the diet. In some instances, modification of dietary habits can be formalized in group therapy programs.

All physicians, nurses, and dietitians who have extensive contact with diabetic patients should be able to determine an individual's daily caloric needs based on ideal body weight and activity. These facts are essential for the construction of a dietary prescription. Once developed, the prescription should permit wide flexibility in the choice of foods.[10]

Specific Diet Proposals

Obese non–insulin-dependent diabetic   For this large group of patients (probably 5 to 7 million in the United States) caloric restriction is the major concept to be conveyed. Moderate weight loss of 10 to 15 lb is often accompanied by improvement in glucose tolerance. Observations such as these have stimulated Davidson and his colleagues to reinstitute the practice of Naunyn and use short-term fasts (one week) as initial diet therapy in obese diabetics. This technique should be started only under close medical supervision and in patients capable of measuring urine ketones and comprehending the possible adverse effects of starvation.[12]

Insulin and oral hypoglycemic agents can often be discarded after patients have lost 5 to 15 lb and before ideal body weight is attained. Protein-sparing diets also induce weight loss in the obese diabetic.[13] The method by which the adipose tissue mass is reduced (and insulin receptor number increased) seems of little relevance; weight loss and improvement in glucose tolerance are what count. Weight loss is ineffective unless maintained. Efforts to achieve ideal body weight should continue; the loss of 1 to 1.5 lb per week indicates that the patient is adhering to a hypocaloric intake.

How much carbohydrate should the obese diabetic consume? Recently, the Committee on Nutrition and Human Needs of the United States Senate suggested a set of national dietary goals (Table 17-2).[14] These goals are applicable to diabetics and nondiabetics alike. While opinion may differ about specifics of these recommendations, the general principles, especially those referrable to dietary carbohydrate, are in line with guidelines issued by the American Diabetes Association in 1971.[15] There is no need to restrict "disproportionately the intake of carbohydrates in the diet of most diabetic patients." Except for that segment of the diabetic population with carbohydrate-induced endogenous hypertriglyceridemia, the carbohydrate component of the diet should comprise 50% to 60% of total calories. These carbohydrates should be mostly in the form of complex polysaccharides such as those in vegetables, bread, and rice. Simple carbohydrates (monosaccharides and disaccharides such as glucose, fructose, and sucrose) should be limited to 15% of the total carbohydrate calories.

Table 17-2
Dietary Goals for the United States

1. Carbohydrate consumption should comprise 55% to 60% of total calories.
2. Reduce refined sugar to 15% of total calories.
3. Fat consumption should comprise 30% of total calories.
   Saturated fats — 10%
   Monounsaturated fats — 10%
   Polyunsaturated fats — 10%
4. Dietary cholesterol should be limited to 300 mg daily.
5. Reduce salt intake to 3.0 gm daily.

Adopted from US Senate Select Committee on Nutritional and Human Needs.[16]

Some continue to contend that carbohydrates, especially refined sugars, are diabetogenic, yet the general consensus is that when nutritional factors are correlated with the prevalence of diabetes in several populations around the world, the "most impressive and consistent association" was between fatness and diabetes, rather than between a specific foodstuff and diabetes.[17]

Obese diabetics should consume at least 15% of their total caloric expenditure as protein. Fat should comprise no more than 35% of total ingested energy. Debate persists about the role of polyunsaturated fats in the pathogenesis of atherosclerosis and abnormal cholesterol metabolism. In the face of uncertainty, diabetics are advised to limit their cholesterol and saturated fat intake in an effort to prevent or delay the macroangiopathy that is such a frequent concomitant of diabetes.

Insulin-dependent diabetics   Youngsters with diabetes must ingest calories in adequate amounts to ensure normal growth rates. Nutritionally sound diets for nondiabetics are equally sound for diabetics. The one caveat is that insulin-requiring diabetics should limit the quantity of refined sugars (monosaccharides and disaccharides) to avoid high postprandial levels of glucose. Whereas it is appreciated that normal subjects have a higher postprandial blood glucose after glucose- or sucrose-containing meals than after a starch meal,[18] no recent comparable data are available for insulin-requiring diabetics. Healthy subjects absorb a glucose-and-starch meal at the same rate.[19]

The most important dietary concept that the insulin-requiring diabetic must grasp pertains to the timing of meals. Most insulin-dependent individuals receive one or two doses of intermediate-acting insulin with or without rapid-acting insulin daily, and hence caloric intake must coincide with the action of the glucose-lowering agent; a regular diet routine is essential. Insulin-taking diabetics must always carry a ready source of simple carbohydrate to counteract hypoglycemia. The division of total daily calories so that fractions of one- or two-tenths are taken at mealtime and one-tenth at a snack is a good standard, but more importantly the dietary pattern must be tailored to fit the individual patient's activity and meal routine.

These simple concepts of dietary management must be presented to the patient and his or her family from the onset of therapy. Young diabetics must recognize the need for balanced meals eaten at regular intervals early in the course of their disease. Failure of pediatricians or other physicians to emphasize these basic principles on early contacts with such patients often results in individuals who are recalcitrant later in life, not only to a reasonable diet approach, but also to a general appreciation of their disease.

Related Issues

While major advancements that help to elucidate the physiology of the beta cell and the pathophysiology of diabetes have been made in the last decade, few practical studies that relate dietary modifications and diabetes have been initiated. For example, it may startle clinicians to know that there is no substantial evidence to demonstrate that sucrose causes more severe hyperglycemia in the insulin-dependent diabetic than equicaloric amounts of complex carbohydrates. Many simple questions that relate diet and diabetics remain unanswered.

Several practical points require emphasis. Most physicians are too busy and have inadequate background to instruct the diabetic properly and continuously about diet.[20] Better use must be made of the educational talents of dietitians and nurses. Employment of meal lists and diets produced by pharmaceutical manufacturers is not an effective way for the physician to meet this challenge.

What about artificial sweeteners? Are they needed by diabetics? Obviously, these substances have no nutritional value. Saccharin and cyclamates are not weight-reducing compounds. Unfortunately, the preference for sweetness is acquired early in life and the habit is difficult to overcome. The only rational argument that can be given for the use of saccharin and cyclamates concerns the psychosocial aspects of a diabetic's life. As physicians, we must have concern for the youngster with diabetes who desires to join peers in social settings where beverages or foods are essential elements. Under such conditions, artificial sweeteners may have a place. Although the carcinogenic potential of saccharin in man seems small, physicians must scrutinize carefully all new information about this relationship. Ideally, the problem will be terminated only when we cease developing a "sweet tooth" early in life.

Summary

Diabetes mellitus is a complex diathesis with two dominant pathogenic lesions: one, a failure of the beta cells of the islet of Langerhans; and the other, a resistance to the actions of insulin. Patients may demonstrate varying degrees of both lesions. Diet therapy has an important place in the treatment of all diabetics. The most important objective of dietary treatment is the control of total caloric intake to attain ideal body weight. Obesity is diabetogenic. Youngsters with diabetes should grow and develop normally; they must eat meals on a regular schedule. Carbohydrate intake should not be disproportionately restricted. Fat intake in diabetics and nondiabetics should comprise only 30% to 35% of total calories. Dietary instruction should not be a one-time affair; physicians should seek the assistance of dietary counselors when they are available. Many basic questions about diet and diabetes remain unanswered.

REFERENCES

1. Siperstein MD: The glucose tolerance test: a pitfall in the diagnosis of diabetes mellitus. *Adv Intern Med* 20:297-323, 1975.

2. Brown JC, Dryburgh JR, Ross SA, et al: Identification and actions of gastric inhibitory polypeptide. *Recent Prog Horm Res* 31:487-532, 1975.

3. Bar RS, Roth J: Insulin receptor status in disease states of man. *Arch Intern Med* 137:474-481, 1977.

4. Goldfine ID: Does insulin need a second messenger? *Diabetes* 26:148-155, 1977.

5. Olefsky JM: The insulin receptor: its role in insulin resistance of obesity and diabetes. *Diabetes* 25:1154-1165, 1976.

6. Fajans SS, Floyd JC Jr, Tattersall RB, et al: The various faces of diabetes in the young. *Arch Intern Med* 136:194-202, 1976.

7. *A Guide for Professionals: The Effective Application of "Exchange Lists for Meal Planning."* New York, American Diabetes Association Inc, and Chicago, The American Dietetic Association, 1977.

8. Cahill GF Jr, Etzweiler DD, Freinkel N: "Control" and diabetes. *N Engl J Med* 294:1004, 1976.

9. Wood FC Jr, Bierman EL: New concepts in diabetic dietetics. *Nutr Today* 7:4-10, 1972.

10. Davidson JK: Controlling diabetes mellitus with diet therapy. *Postgrad Med* 59:115-122, 1976.

11. *Exchange Lists for Meal Planning.* American Diabetes Association Inc, The American Dietetic Association, The National Institute of Arthritis, Metabolism and Digestive Diseases, and National Heart and Lung Institute, 1976.

12. Davidson JK: Plasma glucose lowering effect of caloric restriction in obesity-induced insulin treated diabetes mellitus. *Diabetes* 26(suppl 1):355 (abstract #12), 1977.

13. Bistrian BR, Blackburn GL, Flatt JP, et al: Nitrogen metabolism and insulin requirements in obese diabetic adults on a protein-sparing modified fast. *Diabetes* 25:494-504, 1976.

14. Dietary goals. Editorial. *Lancet* 1:887-888, 1977.

15. Bierman EL, Albrink MJ, Arky RA, et al: Principles of nutrition and dietary recommendations for patients with diabetes mellitus: 1971. *Diabetes* 20:633-634, 1971.

16. Select Committee on Nutritional and Human Needs, US Senate: *Dietary Goals for the United States,* ed 2. Washington, DC, US Government Printing Office, 1977.

17. West KM, Kalbfleisch JM: Influence of nutritional factors on prevalence of diabetes. *Diabetes* 20:99-108, 1971.

18. Crapo PA, Reaven G, Olefsky J: Plasma glucose and insulin responses to orally administered simple and complex carbohydrates. *Diabetes* 25:741-747, 1976.

19. Fogel MR, Gray GM: Starch hydrolysis in man: an intraluminal process not requiring membrane digestion. *J Appl Physiol* 35:263-267, 1973.

20. West KM: Diet therapy of diabetes: an analysis of failure. *Ann Intern Med* 79:425-434, 1973.

18 The Effects of Dietary Components on Brain Function

Steven H. Zeisel, MD

During the last decade effects of nutrition on the brain have been discovered that had previously been unsuspected. The administration of dietary components can predictably cause profound changes in the function of neurons, resulting in alterations in the brain output we call behavior. This is a novel idea, as in the past clinicians believed that meal composition did *not* have an effect on brain function. The brain was thought of as a protected organ, receiving preferential treatment with regard to nutrient supply. In this chapter I shall present evidence that this isolation of the brain is not the case, with respect to three neurotransmitters and their dietary precursors. Animal studies will be presented, establishing the foundation on which clinicians base new therapies for neurologic diseases.

The brain, responsible for control and integration of most functions of the body, is a complex network of billions of neurons. These neurons speak two languages, one electrical and one chemical. Ion fluxes within the neuron generate electrical signals that in turn act to release a chemical signal. These chemicals, called neurotransmitters, diffuse across the

206

synaptic cleft, eventually making contact with receptors on the postsynaptic neuron. Activation of the receptor opens up channels within the membrane of the neuron, ions flow, and an electrical signal is generated in the postsynaptic neuron. At the present time there are perhaps 20 to 30 known compounds that are thought to function as neurotransmitters within the mammalian nervous system. Evidence is accumulating that three types of neurotransmitters, acetylcholine, serotonin, and the catecholamines, are synthesized within neurons in amounts proportional to the availability to the brain of their precursors.[1-3] In each instance the brain content of the precursor can be manipulated by supplementing the diet with large amounts of these precursors.

Dietary Choline and the Biosynthesis of Acetylcholine

Humans normally ingest 100 to 700 mg of choline per day, mostly in the form of the choline-containing compound lecithin (phosphatidylcholine).[4] Lecithin is a part of all membranes, and therefore is found in a wide variety of foods; eggs and liver being especially rich sources (Table 18-1).[4] Once eaten lecithin is metabolized and free choline is contributed to plasma.[5] Plasma choline can double during the course of normal meals,

Table 18-1
Choline and Lecithin Content of Common Foods (mg/100 g Food)

Food	Choline Chloride	Lecithin
Whole milk	5.6	6–10
Cheese	0.0	50–100
Eggs	0.4	394
Calf's liver	650	850
Beef	0.0	453
Ham	0.0	800
Trout	0.0	580
Cauliflower	78	2
Potato	40	1
String beans	21	0.1
Carrots	6–13	5–8
Oatmeal	131	650
Soy bean	237	1480
Wheat germ	0.0	2820
Peanut	0.0	1113
White flour	0.0	346

From Wurtman J: Sources of choline and lecithin in the diet, in Barbeau A, Growdon J, Wurtman J (eds): *Choline and Lecithin in Brain Disorders*. New York, Raven, 1979. With permission.

but it rises even more sharply when lecithin or choline supplements are administered.[5,6]

Transport of choline into the brain is facilitated by a carrier mechanism within the blood-brain barrier that is normally not saturated with choline molecules.[7] Transport of choline from the brain interstitial fluid into the neuron is mediated by two uptake mechanisms, one of which has ample capacity, making this choline available for acetylcholine synthesis. The intraneuronal enzyme choline-acetyltransferase attaches an acetyl-CoA molecule to choline, forming acetylcholine. This enzyme is also unsaturated with respect to choline and, when more choline is made available acetylcholine synthesis is accelerated.[8] In the rat, injection or dietary supplementation with choline elevates acetylcholine concentrations in all brain regions examined (Figure 18-1).[1,9,10]

Increases in the concentration of acetylcholine are not necessarily associated with changes in the quantities of acetylcholine released into the synapse following each nerve impulse. For example, if release were slowed

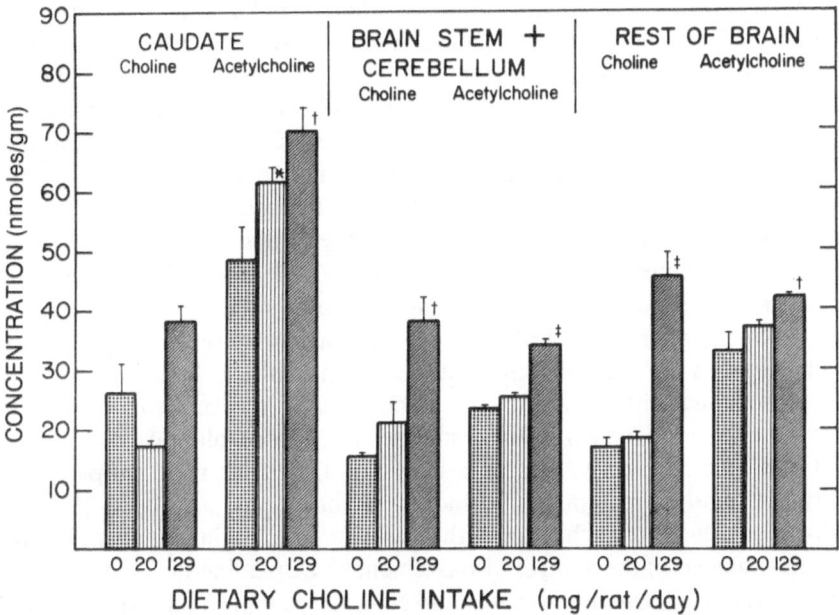

Figure 18-1   Effect of dietary choline content on choline and acetylcholine concentrations in various brain regions. Rats consumed diets having an average of 0, 20, or 129 mg of choline per day for 11 days, consuming 12 ± 1, 11 ± 1, and 7 ± 1 g of food per day, respectively. Bars represent mean concentrations and vertical lines represent the standard error of the mean. "Rest of brain" refers to the cerebrum minus the caudate nucleus. Differences from corresponding rats consuming no choline are indicated by * $P < 0.05$; † $P < 0.01$; ‡ $P < 0.001$. From Cohen E, Wurtman R: Brain acetylcholine synthesis: control by dietary choline. *Science* 191:561–562, 1976. Copyright 1976 by the American Association for the Advancement of Science.

significantly, the ensuing "traffic jam" might result in higher intraneuronal acetylcholine levels. To examine the relationship between precursor and amount of transmitter released, an indirect approach has been necessary, since technical difficulties (eg, isolating specific neurons among billions in the brain or inhibiting the extremely active acetylcholine-degrading enzymes [cholinesterases]) make a direct approach, measuring the number of acetylcholine molecules released, impossible. Release of any neurotransmitter has predictable effects on the postsynaptic neuron, including biochemical changes that are measurable. Neuroanatomists have identified changes that are measurable. They have identified two types of neurons that use acetylcholine as their message; these "speak" to postsynaptic neurons that use catecholamines as their neurotransmitter. The enzyme tyrosine hydroxylase within these postsynaptic neurons increases in activity whenever these neurons' receptors are stimulated by acetylcholine. Thus if choline administration actually causes more acetylcholine to be released, tyrosine hydroxylase should be activated. This increase in activity is indeed measured after choline administration, and it can be prevented by administration of atropine, a drug that blocks the receptors for acetylcholine.[11,12] Increased accumulation of dopamine and its metabolites within these postsynaptic neurons can also be measured after choline administration.[13] Using a preparation of phrenic nerve and diaphragm it has been possible to make direct measurements of acetylcholine molecules released when the nerve is stimulated. When more choline is made available to the nerve there is a proportionate increase in the release of acetylcholine.[14] In slices of brain as well, the availability of choline in the nutrient medium affects the amount of acetylcholine synthesized and released (D. Jenden, personal communication).

Shortly after the first of these basic findings were reported, physicians attempted to use choline in the treatment of neurologic diseases thought to be associated with deficient central cholinergic transmission.[15] Tardive dyskinesia, a movement disorder characterized by involuntary movements of the face and body, is a side effect of treatment with antipsychotic drugs,[16] and is extremely common.[17] It has been postulated that the disorder results from changes in the basal ganglia, brain structures known to be involved in the control of movement.[18] Dopaminergic neurons from the substantia nigra (in the brainstem) enter the caudate nucleus of the basal ganglia and can inhibit a cholinergic neuron, ultimately decreasing inhibition of the motor cortex, resulting in the appearance of unusual movements. After treatment with antipsychotic drugs for a period of time, a phenomenon called hypersensitivity can occur, and the cholinergic neuron becomes more sensitive to inhibition by dopamine. The net result of the disturbance of such finely tuned networks of inhibition and activation is the appearance of unwanted movements, the signs of tardive dyskinesia. If the cholinergic neurons that are still firing, despite the increased inhibition, can be made to release more acetylcholine per impulse, the movements should disappear. Treatment with choline or lecithin has resulted in a marked decrease in the involuntary movements of tardive dyskinesia.[19-21] Effective doses of lecithin (20 g/day of pure phosphatidylcholine) contain more than three times the amount of lecithin eaten in the course of a day in an average human diet. At the present time several manufacturers have made available purified (80% to 95%) lecithin preparations; this contrasts to the "pure" lecithins available at health food stores, which may be only 3% to 20% phosphatidylcholine.

Other clinical applications of choline therapy are still in early stages of investigation. Promising results are being obtained in the treatment of memory disorders,[22,23] and ataxias (balance problems).[24] In the near future data from double-blind studies should be available. The ability to manipulate brain acetylcholine may also be useful in such diseases as mania, Tourette's disease, and other diseases with postulated deficiency of acetylcholine release. This precursor-transmitter relationship may also be extremely important in the healthy developing human, since newborn humans, rats, and rabbits have plasma choline concentrations that are above those seen in adults treated with lecithin or choline.[25]

Tryptophan and Brain Serotonin

Serotonin is a neurotransmitter known to be intimately involved with sleep and analgesia.[26] It is synthesized in neurons from the amino acid tryptophan. The enzyme tryptophan hydroxylase that catalyzes this conversion is unsaturated with respect to tryptophan.[27] Thus when brain tryptophan increases, more serotonin is synthesized (Figure 18-2).[2] Brain tryptophan is ultimately derived from the blood and transported into the brain by a carrier mechanism that is shared by several amino acids, including tryptophan, tyrosine, leucine, isoleucine, valine, and methionine.[28] Tryptophan's share of transport sites is determined by the ratio of tryptophan to the competing neutral amino acids in the blood.[28] Dietary manipulations that alter this ratio, directly alter brain serotonin.[2,29] Administration of tryptophan alone accelerates serotonin synthesis and increases the release of serotonin into the synapse, where it is degraded to form 5-HIAA (Figure 18-2).[2] Diets deficient in tryptophan (eg, corn-based) result in behavioral changes (decreased threshold to pain) associated with decreased brain serotonin.[30] Administration of tryptophan and competing neutral amino acids in a meal may not increase brain serotonin because of competition for entry into the brain; for this reason protein ingestion may not be an optimal way to administer tryptophan.[31] Brain serotonin and tryptophan can, however, be manipulated by the dietary administration of carbohydrate.[29,32] Glucose, via insulin, increases the uptake and metabolism of leucine, isoleucine, and

210

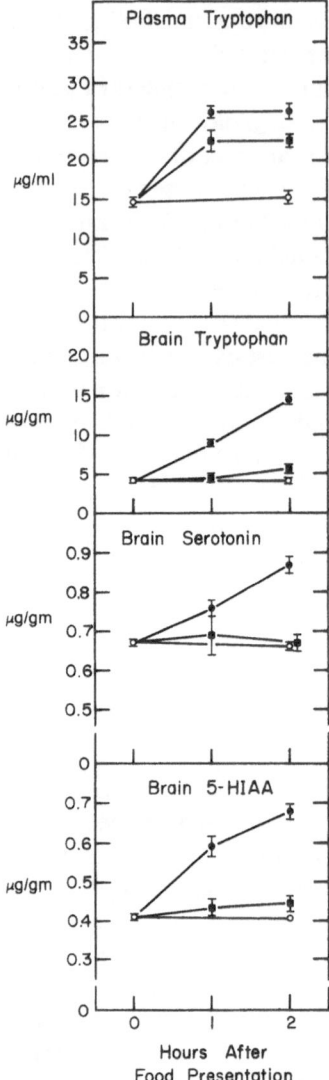

Figure 18-2 Effect of the ingestion of various amino acid-containing diets on plasma and brain tryptophan and brain 5-hydroxyindoles. Groups of eight rats were killed 1 or 2 hours after diet presentation. Vertical bars represent standard errors of the mean. Open circles: fasting controls; closed squares: complete amino acid mixture; closed circles: mixture diet minus tyrosine, phenylalanine, leucine, isoleucine, and valine. The 1- and 2-hour plasma tryptophan concentrations were significantly greater in animals consuming both diets ($P < 0.001$) than in fasting controls. All brain tryptophan, serotonin, and 5-HIAA concentrations were significantly greater in rats consuming the diet lacking the five amino acids than in fasting controls ($P < 0.001$ for all but 1-hour serotonin, $P < 0.01$). From Fernstrom J, Wurtman R: Brain serotonin content: physiological regulation by plasma neutral amino acids. *Science* 178:414–416, 1972. Copyright 1972 by the American Association for the Advancement of Science.

valine by muscle. The net result is a rise in the ratio of tryptophan to the other neutral amino acids, increasing tryptophan transport into the brain.

Untreated rats consuming chow show marked daily variations in plasma tryptophan, with associated changes in brain serotonin.[2] In humans consuming common foods similar variations in plasma tryptophan occur.[33] The physiologic purpose of these changes is not yet known, but it is possible that serotonin neurons in some area of the brain act to monitor tryptophan ingestion. Dietary manipulation of brain serotonin release has been used in the treatment of sleep disorders, and in posthypoxic intention myoclonus.[26,34-36] Five to ten grams of tryptophan administered to normal humans and to insomniacs increased the amount of slow-wave sleep, shortened sleep latency (time to fall asleep), and increased the total minutes of sleep.[26]

Tyrosine and Brain Catecholamines

Catecholamine neurotransmitters (dopamine and norepinephrine) are synthesized from tyrosine, an amino acid ultimately derived from the diet.

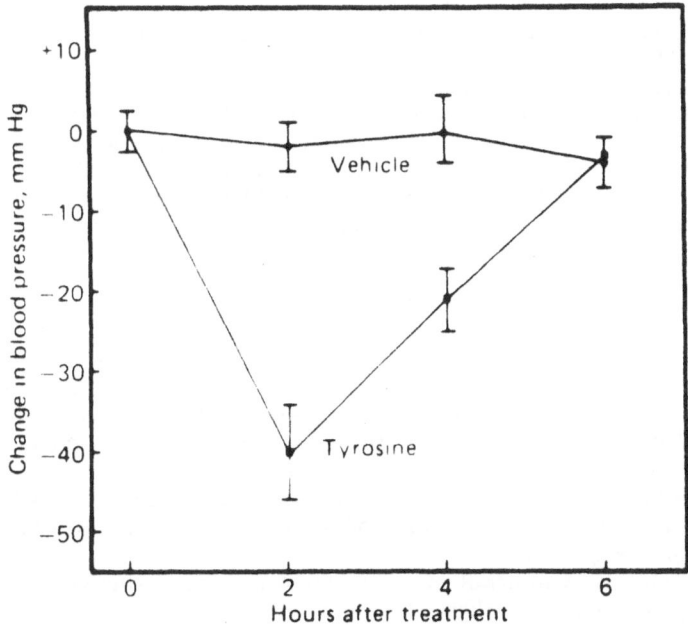

Figure 18-3 Time course of antihypertensive effect of tryosine injection in spontaneously hypertensive rats. Tryosine (200 mg/kg) or vehicle was administered intraperitoneally to groups of six rats. Blood pressures were measured just prior to treatment, and then at two-hour intervals afterward. Data are expressed as change in blood pressure from baseline values (mean ± SEM). The antihypertensive effect of tryosine was significant ($P < 0.01$) at two and four hours. From: Sved et al.[37]

The first step in these biosyntheses is catalyzed by tyrosine hydroxylase, an intraneuronal enzyme that can exist in two forms, activated and inactive. When the enzyme is activated, tryosine availability can be the limiting factor in catecholamine synthesis.[3,13,34] Activation of this enzyme occurs when neurons fire rapidly, as they would when neurons are deficient, eg, in Parkinson's disease, or when postsynaptic receptors are blocked by drugs, eg, in haloperidol administration. Plasma tyrosine, which shares the same blood-brain barrier transport mechanism as tryptophan, reaches the brain in amounts proportional to the ratio of tyrosine to its competitors, the large neutral amino acids.[27] Manipulations that act to increase this ratio (eg, tyrosine administration) increase catecholamine synthesis within brain neurons that are firing rapidly.[3,31,33] Tyrosine administration lowers blood pressure in hypertensive rats (Figure 18-3),[37] and it is likely that tyrosine will be tested in hypertensive humans as well. Preliminary experiments using tyrosine as treatment in Parkinson's disease, depression, and hyperprolactinemia have produced encouraging initial results that warrant further investigation.

REFERENCES

1. Cohen E, Wurtman R: Brain acetylcholine synthesis: control by dietary choline. *Science* 191:561–562, 1976.

2. Fernstrom J, Wurtman R: Brain serotonin content: physiological dependence on plasma tryptophan levels. *Science* 173:149–152, 1971.

3. Gibson C, Wurtman R: Physiological control of brain norepinephrine synthesis by plasma tyrosine concentration. *Life Sci* 22:1399–1406, 1978.

4. Wurtman J: Sources of choline and lecithin in the diet, in Barbeau A, Growdon J, Wurtman R (eds): *Choline and Lecithin in Brain Disorders*. New York, Raven Press, 1979, pp 73–82.

5. Wurtman R, Hirsch M, Growdon J: Lecithin consumption raises serum free choline levels. *Lancet* 2:68–69, 1977.

6. Zeisel S, Growdon J, Wurtman R, et al: Lecithin treatment of tardive dyskinesia: Plasma choline responses to ingested lecithin. *Neurology* (in press).

7. Pardridge W, Cornford E, Braun L, et al: Transport of choline and choline analogues through the blood brain barrier, in Barbeau A, Growdon J, Wurtman R (eds): *Choline and Lecithin in Brain Disorders*. New York, Raven Press, 1979, pp 25–34.

8. White H, Wu J: Kinetics of choline acetyltransferases (E.C.2.3.2.6) from human and other mammalian central and peripheral nervous tissues. *J Neurochem* 20:297–307, 1973.

9. Cohen E, Wurtman R: Brain acetylcholine: increase after systemic choline administration. *Life Sci* 16:1095–1102, 1975.

10. Hirsch M, Growdon J, Wurtman R: Increase in hippocampal acetylcholine following choline administration. *Brain Res* 332:383–385, 1977.

11. Ulus I, Hirsch M, Wurtman R: Trans-synaptic induction of adrenomedullary tyrosine hydroxylase activity by choline. *Proc Natl Acad Sci USA* 74:798–800, 1977.

12. Ulus I, Wurtman R: Choline administration: activation of tryosine hydroxylase in dopaminergic neurons of rats. *Science* 194:1060–1061, 1976.

13. Haubrich D, Gerber N, Pfleuger A: Choline availability and the synthesis of acetylcholine, in Barbeau A, Growdon R, Wurtman R (eds): *Choline and Lecithin in Brain Disorders*. New York, Raven Press, 1979, pp 57–72.

14. Bierkamper G, Goldberg A: Effect of choline on the release of acetylcholine from the neuromuscular junction, in Barbeau A, Growdon J, Wurtman R (eds): *Choline and Lecithin in Brain Disorders*. New York, Raven Press, 1979, pp 243–252.

15. Davis K, Berger P, Hollister L: Choline for tardive dyskinesia. *N Engl J Med* 293:152, 1975.

16. American College of Neuro-Psychopharmacology–FDA Task Force. Neurologic syndromes associated with antipsychotic drug use. *N Engl J Med* 289:20–23, 1973.

17. Jus A, Pineau R, Lachance R, et al: Epidemiology of tardive dyskinesia. *Dis Nerv Syst* 37:210–214, 1976.

18. Baldessarini R: The pathophysiological basis of tardive dyskinesia. *Psychopharmacol Bull* 14:79–81, 1978.

19. Growdon J, Hirsch M, Wurtman R, et al: Oral choline administration to patients with tardive dyskinesia. *N Engl J Med* 297:524–527, 1977.

20. Growdon J, Gelenberg A, Doller J, et al: Lecithin can suppress tardive dyskinesia. *N Engl J Med* 298:1029–1030, 1978.

21. Zeisel S, Gelenberg A, Growdon J, et al: Use of choline and lecithin in the treatment of tardive dyskinesia. *Adv Neuropharmacol* (in press).

22. Etienne P, Gauthier S, Dastoor D, et al: Alzheimer's disease: clinical effects of lecithin treatment, in Barbeau A, Growdon J, Wurtman R (eds): *Choline and Lecithin in Brain Disorders*. New York, Raven Press, 1979, pp 389–398.

23. Christie J, Blackburn I, Glen A, et al: Effects of choline and lecithin on CSF choline levels and on cognitive function in patients with presenile dementia of the Alzheimer type, in Barbeau A, Growdon J, Wurtman R (eds): *Choline and Lecithin in Brain Disorders*. New York, Raven Press, 1979, pp 377–388.

24. Barbeau A: Lecithin in movement disorders, in Barbeau A, Growdon J, Wurtman R (eds): *Choline and Lecithin in Brain Disorders*. New York, Raven Press, 1979, pp 263–272.

25. Zeisel S, Epstein M, Wurtman R: Elevated choline concentration in neonatal plasma. *Life Sci* 26:1827–1831, 1980.

26. Hartman E: L-tryptophan: effects on sleep. *Monogr Neural Sci* 3:26–32, 1976.

27. Pardridge W: Regulation of amino acid availability to brain, in Wurtman R, Wurtman J (eds): *Nutrition and the Brain,* vol 1. New York, Raven Press, 1977, pp 141–204.

28. Fernstrom J, Wurtman R: Brain serotonin content: increase following ingestion of a carbohydrate diet. *Science* 174:1023–1025, 1971.

29. Fernstrom J, Larin F, Wurtman R: Correlations between brain tryptophan and plasma neutral amino acids following food consumption in rats. *Life Sci* 13:517–524, 1973.

30. Fernstrom J, Wurtman R: Elevation of plasma tryptophan by insulin in the rat. *Metabolism* 21:337–342, 1972.

31. Scally M, Wurtman R: Brain tyrosine levels control striatal dopamine synthesis in haloperidol treated rats. *J Neural Transm* 41:1–6, 1977.

32. Fernstrom J, Arnold M, Wurtman R, et al: Diurnal variations in normal and cirrhotic subjects: effect of protein consumption. *J Neur Transm* 14(suppl):133–142, 1978.

33. Wurtman R, Larin F, Mostafapour S, et al: Brain catechol synthesis: control by brain tyrosine concentration. *Science* 185:183–184, 1974.

214

34. Wyatt R, Engelman K, Kupfer D, et al: Effects of L-tryptophan (a natural sedative) on human sleep. *Lancet* 2:842–846, 1970.

35. Oswald I, Ashcroft G, Berger R, et al: Experiments in the chemistry of normal sleep. *Br J Psychiatry* 112:391–399, 1966.

36. De Lean J, Richardson J, Hornykiewicz O: Beneficial effects of serotonin precursors in postanoxic action myoclonus. *Neurology* 26:863–868, 1976.

37. Sved A, Fernstrom J, Wurtman R: Tyrosine administration reduces blood pressure and enhances brain norepinephrine release in spontaneously hypertensive rats. *Proc Natl Acad Sci USA* 76:3511–3514, 1979.

216

cow's milk and, 23
fat in, 22
host resistant factors in, 31–32
preference for, 59

Necrotizing enterocolitis (NEC), 25
 precipitating factors in, 25
Neurotransmitters, 205–206, 211–212
Niacin deficiency, 193
Norepinephrine, 211
Nutrients
 diversion of, 102–104
 overutilization of, 101–102
 sequestration of, 103–104
Nutrient loss
 absolute, 100–101
 functional, 101–104
 infection-induced nutrient loss, 100
Nutrition
 assessment of, in children, 77
 controversies in, 3
 factors involved in, 78
Nutritional excesses, 73
Nutritional management, 93–95

Obesity, 4
Obesity, surgery for
 complications of, 147–151
 historical considerations of, 143–144
 indications for, 144–145
 long-term effects of, 150–151
 morbidity, 148–151
 mortality, 147–148
Olson, 4
Osteoporosis, 119

Parkinson's disease, 212
Pellagra, 4, 18
Phosphate, 101
Phosphorus, 108, 109
Pickwickian syndrome, 146
Potassium, 101, 194
 foods with high, 149
 ^{40}K counting, 154
Poverty, infant mortality and, 59
Primiparas, 66

self-concept of in breast/bottle
 feeding, 68
Progesterone, 119
Protein, 58, 90–92, 102
 binding, 32, 34
 biosynthesis of, 193
 diets, 94, 200
Prothrombin, 134–135
 biosynthesis of, 137–139
 liver, 135–137
 plasma, 135

Rickets, 4
Recommended Dietary Allowances
 (RDA), 18
RNA, 92

Salt (NaCl), 14–15, 58, 193
Scurvy, 4, 18
Serotinin, 206, 209–211
Smoking, 171
Solid foods, infants and, 56
Sugar, 13–14
Sulfur, 101

Tardive dyskinesia, 208–209
T cell, 83, 86, 87, 90, 91
Testosterone, 119
Trace metal deficiencies, 170, 194
Tryptophan, 209–211
Tuberculosis, 73
Tumor systems, 190–191
Tyrosine, 64, 211–212

Vitamin A, 93
Vitamin C, 56
 antihistamine effects of, 1
Vitamin D, 51, 52, 90, 108, 109,
 111–114, 123, 126
Vitamin deficiencies, 169
Vitamin E, 56
Vitamin K
 -dependent carboxylation, 137–139
 structures of, 131

Weight, ideal, 9–11, 200

Zinc, 39, 101, 194